Macrobiotic

Community

Cookbook

Other Avery books about macrobiotics:

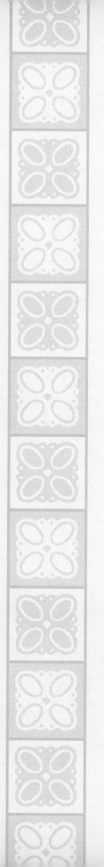

Macrobiotic Community Cookbook

Andrea Bliss-Lerman

Avery • a member of Penguin Group (USA) Inc. • New York

a member of
Penguin Group (USA) Inc.
375 Hudson Street
New York, NY 10014
www.penguin.com

Copyright © 1989, 2003 by Andrea Bliss-Lerman
Christina Pirello's recipe for Sweet Parsnip Soup with Hazelnut Pesto is taken from *Glow: A Prescription for Radiant Health and Beauty* (HPBooks, 2001) and is used with permission.
Illustrations by Vicki Hudon

Library of Congress Cataloging-in-Publication Data

Bliss-Lerman, Andrea.
Macrobiotic community cookbook / Andrea Bliss-Lerman.—[Rev. and updated ed.]
p.   cm.
Includes index.
ISBN 1-58333-165-4
1. Macrobiotic diet—Recipes.   I. Title.
RM235.L47   2003   2003052315
641.5'63—dc21

Printed in the United States of America
3   5   7   9   10   8   6   4   2

Book design by Meighan Cavanaugh

Contents

Preface

More and more people are becoming aware that a low-fat, low-sugar, high-fiber diet is beneficial. The macrobiotic lifestyle includes a diet that is not only low in fat and sugar and high in fiber—it includes so much more! It encompasses every facet of life. For health does not simply mean physical well-being. It also incorporates self-esteem, spiritual beliefs, and outlook on life.

There are two things that those who follow the macrobiotic way seek: One is balance, and the other is an appreciation for all that they have. Through study, application, and experimentation in macrobiotics, I have found that these aspirations can be reached. I have been able to find a great balance within myself through this lifestyle, and now recognize the effects that foods have on my personality and how I relate to myself and to other people.

The foods that people eat become part of them, and creating a total balance in each meal can be a practical, positive step toward creating a balance in all aspects of life. Health and happiness go hand in hand—as individuals become healthier within themselves, they are able to touch the lives of others in a way that sparks an interest in physical, mental, and spiritual health. They can also encourage others to seek a more peaceful way of life. As one person reaches out and touches another, the next person does the same, and eventually, a healthier and more peaceful world is created for all.

I thought that a cookbook that included contributions from the macrobiotic community was a good idea, because the idea of a "community" is one of balance and harmony. After I decided to write this book, I sent letters to people in the macrobiotic community, asking them to contribute recipes. I received a generous number of replies and supportive letters.

I had the delightful opportunity to meet Wendy Esko, who has written many books on macrobiotic cooking philosophy. Meeting Wendy and casually chatting about the book was a special experience for me.

Cornellia Aihara of the George Ohsawa Macrobiotic Foundation–Vega Study Center sent a wonderful chapati recipe. Natural food store owners, macrobiotic counselors, restaurant owners, and people who run macrobiotic centers all over the country have shared their warmth, interest, and support. I truly appreciate the time, effort, and desire it took for each one of them to become a part of my book.

My own recipes were compiled over a period of about three years, as I cooked for people who were trying to recover from serious illnesses, people simply interested in incorporating macrobiotic-style cookery into their own repertoire of recipes, and friends and family members who just like the taste of good food. Over the years I have modified a few of the recipes, and these changes are included in this edition. Some changes are due to personal preference, and others to the availability of commercial products.

Macrobiotic Community Cookbook can be an effective contribution to the number of macrobiotic cookbooks that line bookstore shelves. The recipes are mostly Western in their approach, and many are appropriate for, or can be easily adjusted for, people on healing diets. Devising new recipes, and cooking and sharing them, can be enjoyable and fulfilling as you take the challenge of finding your own personal balance through ever-changing and ever-growing experiences. With a basic knowledge and awareness of what balance is all about and how to achieve it, you may gain greater control of your life. If this book can inspire a few people to reach out, take the plunge, and attempt to become healthier and happier through macrobiotics, then one main purpose has been achieved.

I would like to thank all the people who generously contributed their recipes and personal information to the book. I would like to thank my best friend and husband, Larry. Without his support and love, this book probably would not have become a reality. I would like to thank all the people who taught us about macrobiotics and the positive effects of community and balance in eating, relationships, and life. It has been a privilege to incorporate many of the macrobiotic teachings into my life with Larry. Our mutual desire for wholeness, health, and peace inside of ourselves, as well as outside, has greatly contributed to the fertile soil of our lives from which wonderful things have been able to grow. I am even grateful for the hard lessons we learned along the way and how companioning each other on this macrobiotic journey has transformed and blessed us as individuals and as a marital couple.

Thanks also to my three daughters, Elizabeth, Jessica, and Stephanie, who each in her own way, unknowingly and often with childlike wisdom, made significant impacts on this book.

I would like to extend a very special thanks to Stephen Blauer, Rudy Shur, and Karen Heffernan from Avery, and my editor Kristen Jennings from the offices of Penguin. Their encouragement, patience, and assistance helped make this book come to life. Thank you, George and Lima Ohsawa, Michio and Aveline Kushi, and Herman and Cornelia Aihara, for spreading macrobiotics in order to create "one peaceful world," and for allowing me to make one small contribution to your dream.

Andrea Bliss-Lerman

Foreword

In the past, communities were often defined by space. They were composed mostly of people who lived near one another: friends, neighbors, and members of one's extended family. The kinship, sense of belonging, and support provided by one's family and neighboring community were and still are an essential part of our existence.

Today, with modern transportation and instant communication, communities extend far beyond the boundaries of immediate geography. They are no longer being defined by space but more by shared dreams and aspirations.

Over the last twenty years, the macrobiotic community has grown to become global. Macrobiotic families and friends live on every continent. Like the members of a planetary extended family, they share a similar way of eating and a common dream of health and peace for all humanity.

In this book you will meet some of the members of this worldwide community. As you will see in the recipes, their cooking styles are as diverse and varied as the individuals themselves. The principle of macrobiotics—yin and yang, or the universal laws of harmony and balance—underlies the approach to food and cooking presented here. Since this principle is one of constant change and adaptation, it is essential to consider unique climatic, seasonal, and individual differences when we cook. The recipes in this book illustrate this principle of change, and are reflections of the individual circumstances and preferences of each of the contributors.

Many of the friends who contributed recipes to *Macrobiotic Community Cookbook* studied at the Kushi Institute in Boston or were influenced by the style of cooking taught there. At the KI we teach the importance of adapting macrobiotic principles to each person's needs. For example, someone seeking to recover from illness would need to be more careful about the foods he selects than someone in good health who is making a gradual transition to a naturally balanced diet. Because the recipes in this book represent a more gradual, transitional approach to macrobiotic cooking, not all the ingredients are appropriate for those with health problems. In many cases, these are indicated in the recipes. Dietary guidelines and recipes for health recovery are presented in books such a *Aveline Kushi's Complete Guide to Macrobiotic Cooking* and *The Macrobiotic Cancer Prevention Cookbook*.

I would like to thank Andrea Bliss-Lerman for her patient efforts in contacting our friends and compiling the recipes contained in these pages. I invite you to try these delicious natural food dishes, and regardless of where you live, join the growing community of friends throughout the world who are creating health and peace with the foods they cook each day.

Wendy Esko
Clinton, Michigan

Introduction

WHAT IS MACROBIOTICS?

Macrobiotics means "great life." It is a philosophy that enables people to create a physical, mental, and spiritual balance for ultimate health and happiness. Physical balance can be created by eating foods that are appropriate for your personal environmental conditions. This is a cookbook, so, obviously, food will be emphasized—but it should be noted that macrobiotics is not only a diet; it is a way of life.

George Ohsawa is the first man credited with defining and spreading macrobiotics as it applies to daily life. One of Ohsawa's students, Michio Kushi, began teaching macrobiotics to a small group of people who were eager to learn about natural health. As more and more people became interested, Michio Kushi and his wife, Aveline, published several books and lectured all over the world. When they saw a need for a source of natural foods, the Kushis opened a store called Erewhon, and to educate others about macrobiotics, they founded the East West Foundation and the Kushi Institute (both educational nonprofit organizations) and started the *East West Journal* (a monthly publication that features the macrobiotic lifestyle). Mr. and Mrs. Kushi have enlightened many about the importance of living physically, mentally, and spiritually in harmony with nature. Their work has been an invaluable contribution to the total health of millions.

Herman and Cornellia Aihara, two more of George Ohsawa's students who came to the United States from Japan, taught macrobiotics for a number of years in California, where they founded the George Ohsawa Macrobiotic Foundation. Herman was a philosopher, scientist, engineer, and teacher. In his passion to spread the knowledge of macrobiotics, he became a prolific writer of articles and books. Cornellia is an accomplished teacher of macrobiotic cooking, philosophy, child care, and natural home remedies. Motivated by a deep sense of purpose and calling, Herman and Cornellia have traveled throughout the United States and Europe giving lectures and cooking classes.

The macrobiotic diet changes for different people in different environments, and at different stages in life. However, there are some basic food combinations that most people would consider to be "macro." Whether labeled as belonging to this philosophy or not, the foods on this diet are wholesome, nutritious, natural foods—many of which our ancestors, who never heard of macrobiotics, ate regularly.

Food contains vitamins and minerals, but it also contains an intangible energy. This energy is what gives all things life—it is a life force, or life's essence. For a macrobiotic diet, it has been recommended that half of what you eat each day consist of grain. Whole grain contains all this energy within its compact seed. The energy force of cracked and ground grains is dispersed by the process of cracking or grinding, so it is not as strengthening as grain in its whole form. This does not mean that fragmented grains should be avoided; it means that most people could achieve greater health if flour products such a bread, cookies, noodles, and cake did not comprise the major portion of their grain intake.

Vegetables make up about 35 percent of your daily fare on a macrobiotic diet. Locally grown produce, or produce that is suitable to be grown in your region, is stressed as helping you to be better adapted to your climate—just as that plant is. In other words, a diet in a temperate climate would be more balanced if it were centered on fruits and vegetables from that region, rather than on imported tropical produce, such a mangos and bananas, on a daily basis.

Vegetables can be eaten raw, pickled, baked, boiled, steamed, sautéed, broiled, or fried. They may be eaten plain or seasoned, in grain or bean dishes, in soups or stews, or in a variety of other ways.

The rest of the macrobiotic diet consists of beans, bean products, sea vegetables, nuts, seeds, fish, fruit, and desserts.

All foods, and the ways they are cooked or prepared, have certain qualities that affect the body in specific ways. Length of cooking time, amount of heat, amount of salt, and different cutting techniques provide ways to vary food and its qualities. Changing cooking styles contributes to the nourishment of the diverse types of energies within our bodies, and makes food interesting and appealing.

MACROBIOTIC COOKING

The macrobiotic style of cookery is based on traditional principles and values. It uses only natural, fresh foods and traditional cooking methods.

After reading this book and trying the recipes, you will see that the variety of basic foods is great. The many different ways of preparing, seasoning, and presenting foods provide unlimited opportunities for creating your own irresistible dishes. The food tastes great, and you will find that you are healthier and happier. What could be better? I find it exciting, and I'm sure you will, too.

Because this type of cooking involves more thought, time, and energy than fast-food cookery, more of the cook's feelings and energy is transmitted into the food. Though this may seem rather abstract, a meal prepared by someone who enjoys cooking will taste much better, and feel better inside, than a meal prepared by someone who dislikes and resents cooking. It is important to realize that cooking can be a means of "giving of yourself" in order to help those you cook for become better balanced within themselves. The happier and healthier they are, the more they are able to influence other people to become happier, and it goes on from there.

Looking at the larger picture, you cannot help but see that healthful, balanced cookery, even on a small scale within your home, can affect many people and be instrumental in helping to create a happier world. Cooking for a family or friends is a much more important job than many people realize, and should be done with knowledge and care to create health, happiness, and satisfaction. Natural cookery realizes the importance of balanced, whole foods, and how the use of these foods influences those you cook for. Now let's look at some specific foods and kitchen equipment used in whole-foods cookery.

BASIC FOODS

Organically grown foods have been grown without chemical insecticides, on soil that has been free from chemical fertilizers for a certain number of years. Organically grown grains, beans, vegetables, and fruits are superior in quality and taste to the mass-produced foods sold in most supermarkets. Whenever possible, purchase organically grown foods. The use of preservative-free food, which is devoid of artificial additives and colorings, is a major step toward creating a healthier diet.

GRAINS

Whole grain entrées can be prepared from any of the following: barley, brown rice (short grain, medium grain, long grain, sweet rice), buckwheat, corn, millet, oats, rye, and wheat. Other whole grains that are used less often are quinoa and triticale.

On a macrobiotic diet, properly prepared whole grains constitute half of your daily portion of food. They provide necessary vitamins and minerals, fiber, and a slow-burning source of energy. Glass jars provide wonderful storage containers for keeping grains.

Before they are cooked, grains should be thoroughly cleaned of any dust, sticks, or little stones. One way of doing this is to put the grain in a pot, cover it with tap water, and swirl the water and grain together with your hand. Discard the cloudy water into the sink. Do this about three times, removing any debris that may have come out of hiding when you swirled the water. If the grain is particularly dirty, rinse it several times until it is clean.

After cleaning the grain, you may prepare it in a number of ways. It can be pressure-cooked, baked, sprouted, boiled, or roasted and then boiled. It can be seasoned with salt only, or with numerous other seasonings. Grains may be cooked with vegetables, condiments, sea vegetables, beans, seeds, or other grains.

Whole-grain brown rice is one of the most versatile grains. Its sweet, nutty flavor combines well with other grains and vegetables. It can be purchased in the form of short grain, medium grain, long grain, and glutinous sweet rice. Each type has its own unique flavor and properties.

Short- and medium-grain rice are good, basic grains for everyday use. Long-grain rice provides an interesting texture when combined with short-grain rice, and a pleasant variation when prepared by itself. It is especially welcome in warm weather, as it has a cooling effect on the body. Sweet, glutinous rice is higher in fat and protein than the other varieties. After cooking, it is very sticky, and lends itself well to making rich, puffed-rice cakes called mochi and to puréeing in a food processor or pounding in a suribachi to achieve a stretchy, melted-cheese–like consistency. Its higher fat and protein content, as well as its unique consistency, makes sweet rice a wonderful food for children and pregnant women.

Most of the grains listed here can be enjoyed alone, or as cereals, soups, or entrées. Whole rye and wheat, in my opinion, are much more palatable either sprouted or eaten in small amounts, cooked with rice. To cook with rice, soak the rye or wheat in water overnight, combine with rice, and then either pressure-cook or boil. These whole grains will add a delightful, chewy texture to the rice.

Grain products such as noodles, flours, seitan, rice cakes, sourdough bread, muffins, crackers, and cookies help round out the grain category with their unique textures, flavors, and familiarity. With these foods, the possibilities of creating copies of certain dishes that were enjoyed in your premacrobiotic days, and of creating new recipes, are almost endless.

Beans

Dried beans and bean products contribute a concentrated source of protein, along with B vitamins, iron, and calcium. Combined with grains, the quality of their protein is superior to animal foods, as their fat content is very low and their fiber and mineral contents are high. Chickpeas, lentils, and azuki beans are the basic bean choices to be used most of the time. However, black soybeans, black turtle beans, kidney beans, lima beans, navy beans, pinto beans, split peas, and others offer even more of an opportunity for growth in the area of creative cookery. Dried beans, like grains, keep well in tightly covered glass jars. Beans are delicious, and are easily digested by most people if cooked properly.

There are several methods of cooking beans that increase their digestibility. First, rinse the beans in a strainer, removing any stones, sticks, and spoiled beans. (It is hard to enjoy a bowl of luscious bean soup when you keep chomping on tiny stones and sticks!) Then, you can choose any of the following ways of preparing dried beans to make them easier to digest.

- Cook them with kombu or kombu and bay leaf.
- Boil them rapidly for about ten minutes before pressure-cooking or pot cooking.
- Soak them overnight and discard the excess soaking water.
- Season them with miso.
- Serve them with some sort of pickled vegetable.

Individuals with digestive problems may have to experiment to find out which method is suitable for their specific needs.

Beans may be combined with grains, vegetables, sea vegetables, and seeds. You will discover just how versatile beans are when you make them into soups, burgers, loaves, dips, sandwich spreads, and croquettes.

Bean products such as tofu (fresh and dried), tempeh, miso, tamari, and natto beans are also integral parts of the macrobiotic diet. They provide even more of an opportunity for inventiveness and variation in cooking.

Tofu, which is pressed soybean curd, is an especially unique food. The nature of tofu gives it an incredible ability to be a chewy-textured side dish with a meatlike consistency; a scrambled-egg substitute; or a rich and creamy white sauce or creamed soup. The bland flavor of tofu will absorb any seasonings one may decide to use, so it is quite a versatile food.

VEGETABLES

The use of vegetables in whole-foods cookery is a special category that deserves more time and attention than it is usually given in standard American cuisine. Locally and organically grown produce is preferable. Leafy greens such as collards, kale, watercress, carrot tops, turnip greens, and bok choy add a light feeling and bright quality to any meal. This is especially so when these greens are steamed for only a few minutes. Steaming them enhances their color, rather than washing it out.

It is important to wash greens very carefully to remove any sand, dirt, or little critters that may be clinging to the leaves. A good way of doing this is to separate the leaves and place them in a large bowl of water. Wash each leaf separately, carefully removing any unwanted particles or guests. The greens are now ready to be eaten in a raw salad, or steamed, boiled, or sautéed.

Ground vegetables, such as winter squash, cauliflower, and pumpkin, are eaten often in almost all styles and combinations of vegetable cookery. Soups, stews, grain and vegetable dishes, vegetable platters, pickles, and desserts are just a few samplings of the uses of ground vegetables.

To clean ground vegetables, scrub the skins well with a vegetable brush, peeling off and discarding any discolored or spoiled-looking sections of the peel. For certain dishes, you may decide to peel the vegetables anyway. Of course, cauliflower need not be peeled. Simply rinse it under cool tap water.

Stem and root vegetables offer stable, strengthening energy and a feeling of being "anchored." Carrots, burdock, parsnips, daikon, onions, radishes, rutabagas, and turnips can be prepared with the same degree of variety as ground vegetables. Thoroughly scrub them with a vegetable brush before using, and discard any off-color sections of the peel. Onions and waxed rutabagas are always peeled.

Pickled Vegetables

Pickled vegetables are eaten toward the end of a meal to aid digestion and assimilation of foods. Carrot slices, onion slices, cauliflowerets, broccoli flowerets, daikon slices, cucumber slices, green beans, green pepper slices, red radishes, turnip slices, and cabbage slices all make delicious pickles.

Basic, quick pickles are made either by pressing them with salt; layering them in a salty brine made from either half water and half salt, half water and half tamari, or half water and half umeboshi vinegar; or by pressing thin slices of vegetables into a keg of miso. These take from eight to twenty-four hours to pickle. Variations on pickle recipes may include herbs, spices, rice vinegar, and sweeteners. Lengths of pickling times can also be varied.

Sea Vegetables

Unlike many other "healthful" diets, macrobiotics presents individuals with a food that some people find strange at first taste. Sea vegetables, or seaweeds, as they are often called, supply an invaluable source of concentrated minerals and vitamin B_{12}. They have a powerful healing capacity and strengthening ability, making them a much-needed food by many people today.

Sea vegetables are usually purchased in a dried form and can last for years in a bag on a kitchen shelf. The ones used are hijiki, arame, wakame, nori, kombu, and agar-agar. Each one has its own unique flavor, texture, and smell. They may be eaten as side dishes, in soups, in salads, combined with beans and/or grains, and in desserts. Even tempting appetizers can be created using these wonderful vegetables from the sea. Please note: sometimes cats find the flavor and aroma of certain sea vegetables irresistible. I found out—the hard way—that cooked hiziki left on the kitchen counter may become a feast for a family cat.

FISH

Fresh fish and seafood can be enjoyed once or twice a week by those on a macrobiotic diet. White-fleshed fish may be eaten on a regular basis by people who are in good health, while other types of fish and shellfish may be eaten less often. Broiling, baking, pan-frying, and poaching are all excellent ways of preparing fish. Deep-fried fish and fish soup can also be incorporated into one's repertoire of fish recipes.

Try to buy fish that is as fresh as possible. Most of the time, if it has a fishy smell, it is not fresh. I try to buy fish the same day I plan to cook it (unless it needs an overnight marinade, in which case it would be purchased the day before). After purchasing it, I store the fish in the refrigerator until just before I cook it. Fish lends itself well to being seasoned with lemon, tamari, and herbs such as garlic, ginger, and dill.

FRUIT

Ah, the delectable taste of fresh fruit eaten raw or cooked in desserts! This is a part of whole-foods cookery that many people look forward to. Although macrobiotics, as practiced in a temperate climate, is not based on large amounts of fruit, fruit does have its place in desserts, snacks, garnishes, and salad fixings, such as in my Waldorf Salad Variation. In temperate climates, the winter supply of locally grown and stored fruit is limited to apples, pears, and dried fruit. A greater variety of fruit is available in the summer. Melons, peaches, nectarines, apricots, grapes, berries, cherries, and plums are all appropriate summer choices for people in temperate climates.

NUTS AND SEEDS

Nuts and seeds may be used as garnishes, condiments, snacks, appetizers, or dessert ingredients. Sesame, pumpkin, and sunflower seeds are used regularly. Sesame is especially popular as a garnish or condiment and puréed sesame seeds make a seed butter called tahini. Tahini is of Middle Eastern origin and is made from lightly roasted or raw hulled sesame seeds ground to a paste. It is usually unsalted. Sesame butter is prepared from unhulled sesame seeds that are roasted and ground to a paste with the addition of sea salt. Both of them should be used sparingly, as they are very rich and oily. Besides being sources of oil, seeds are also excellent sources of iron and calcium.

Nuts, too, constitute a small percentage of the macrobiotic diet. They can be used interchangeably with seeds in recipes. A small amount of roasted nuts can transform a plain dessert into a special treat. The most commonly used nuts are almonds, pecans, walnuts, chestnuts, and peanuts.

OILS AND CONDIMENTS

Oils and condiments can help change an ordinary meal into an exciting, unique experience. Since macrobiotic cookery generally avoids the use of heavy spices and seasonings, variations in flavor are achieved by using natural seasonings, and altering cooking styles and cutting techniques.

Macrobiotic cooking chooses the "gentle" approach. Foods are carefully prepared and delicately seasoned to enhance their natural flavors—not overpower them. Unrefined sesame oil, dark and light, and unrefined corn oil are the most commonly used oils. Sesame is used more in grain and vegetable preparations, and corn is used more for desserts. I also enjoy using olive oil, especially in salad dressings. The unrefined oils are so rich-tasting and flavorful that I have decided to include them with the seasonings. Small amounts can be used to add a rich quality to any dish.

Some of the standard condiments and seasonings used in macrobiotic cooking include ginger, sesame salt (roasted sesame seeds and salt ground together), umeboshi plums, tekka (a roasted vegetable and miso condiment), brown rice vinegar, miso, tamari, natural mustard, mirin, and sea salt.

Miso and tamari are both soy-based products made from fermented soybeans. Miso is very rich in digestion-promoting enzymes, protein, and vitamin B_{12}, making it an almost irreplaceable food for people following the macrobiotic diet. It is rarely, if ever, boiled, as boiling destroys the live enzymes that are so important. That is why I recommend buying unpasteurized miso. Simmering miso in soup, rather than boiling it, is the preferable method of preparation. Tamari, another commonly used seasoning, has a rich, salty taste. Either of these can change a dull, pale soup into a rich, full-bodied broth, for example, though their usage is not limited to soups. Stews, salads, vegetables, beans, fish, and sea vegetables can all be enhanced by the addition of miso or tamari.

Sea salt is the preferable choice when considering daily salt in cooking because, unlike common table salt, it is unrefined, free from chemical additives, and contains some trace minerals.

You will see or may have seen the word *kuzu* mentioned in some of the recipes. Kuzu is a white, chunky starch made from the root of the kuzu plant. It is used as a thickener instead of cornstarch. However, unlike cornstarch, kuzu is very strengthening and is also used in various medicinal preparations.

BEVERAGES

What do macrobiotic people drink if they don't drink those well-known soft drinks, tropical fruit juices, and cow's milk? To some people it seems as though there is nothing left!

The most important liquid used is spring or well water. Almost everything is cooked with water, and pure, nonchemicalized water is essential for good health. Health aside, it tastes better and helps the food it is cooked with taste better. The use of distilled water is discouraged because distilled water is considered to be "dead" water. All the minerals and life energy have been removed from it. Spring or well water still contains minerals and that intangible life energy, but lacks the harmful additives that permeate many of the tap waters now available to us.

Besides water, some of the common beverages used are bancha tea, grain coffee, barley tea, amasake, sparkling water, and apple juice or cider made with spring or well water. Since so many of the foods on this diet contain a great deal of liquid, either naturally or through the addition of water in the cooking process, it isn't necessary to consume large quantities of beverages. A cup of tea after meals is usually sufficient for most people. However, there are always exceptions, and if a person is engaged in heavy physical labor or exercise that produces a great deal of perspiration and thirst, then that person should drink more liquid.

NO DAIRY?

Since dairy products are concentrated sources of saturated fat, highly mucus forming, and a common allergen, they are not recommended as standard foods on the macrobiotic diet. In their book, *The Macrobiotic Way,* Michio Kushi and Stephen Blauer explain:

> *Research by the National Academy of Sciences . . . has linked the fats in dairy products to an increase in the presence of cysts and tumors of the breasts, uterus, and ovaries in American women. In addition, many people find that dairy foods cause the body to produce excess mucus, which often appears as a postnasal drip, symptoms of allergies, breathing difficulties, and blockage or irritation of the sinuses. The minimal use or complete avoidance of dairy foods has, in many cases, caused a reversal of these and other related problems.*

Dr. Frank Oski's book entitled *Don't Drink Your Milk* is still an eye-opener regarding the intake of milk products and their effect on the human body. Dr. Oski was a noted and well-respected pediatrician who wrote this book many years ago when many people in the medical community were virtually unaware of the role of dietary choices in curing and preventing health problems.

As society has become increasingly aware of healthy living and eating, dairy products no longer carry the stamp of calcium perfection that they once had. Milk is no longer seen as the "perfect food." My three daughters have grown to be strong, healthy young women since the first printing of this book, and their dairy intake has been minimal. My daughters were given the knowledge and freedom to make wise food choices inside and outside of the home. As they became older and more independent, their food preferences often reflected those of advertising and their peers rather than our home. However, I am certain that the whole-foods diet that helped to nourish and nurture each one of them was an invaluable gift to their bodies, minds, and spirits.

At this time in our culture, commercial nondairy substitute foods and meat substitutes abound in supermarkets and health food stores across the country. Calcium-fortified soy milk, rice milk, almond milk, and oat milk are available. You can buy soy yogurt, soy cheese, rice cheese, soy meat alternatives, and dairy-free frozen desserts. Most of these may be enjoyable additions to standard macrobiotic fare and easily incorporated into a standard macrobiotic diet. For those on specific healing diets, it would be wise to contact a trained macrobiotic nutritional counselor when deciding whether or not to expand your personal dietary plan. For healthy children and adults, many of these commercial products, taken in moderation, are welcome treats and offer a bit more flexibility to food preparation and the diet in general.

As I speak about dairy and commercial substitutes, I am also aware that there is a sizable segment of the population who struggles with gluten sensitivity or wheat-related allergies. Gluten is found in wheat, oats, barley, and rye. Substitutions for wheat and gluten products are commercially available in supermarkets, health food stores, Asian markets, and by mail order to specific stores that specialize in providing gluten-free products. There are several brands of wheat-free and gluten-free flours, noodles, crackers, and cookies. Rice noodles may be substituted for wheat noodles in any of these recipes. You may have to experiment to find the brand of rice noodles most agreeable to your taste. There is a variety on the market. Soft and sticky, but not watery, short-grain rice or sweet rice sweetened with rice syrup or maple syrup and a couple of tablespoons of nut butter may be used as a flourless, gluten-free, wheat-free piecrust in place of the couscous crust that is suggested in two of the recipes in this book. With a touch of imagination and mindfulness, it is possible to alter the standard macrobiotic recommendations to accommodate gluten-free and wheat-free diets in ways that produce satisfying daily fare and creative dishes for special occasions.

STOCKING THE KITCHEN

Stocking and organizing your kitchen may seem like an insurmountable task when you first decide to change over to a whole-foods diet. I would suggest that you do things gradually, so that you enjoy the changeover and it doesn't become a burden. Below is a starter cooking utensil and equipment list that will be helpful. As time goes on and you are cooking more, you may find it necessary to add to this list.

The best-quality pots and pans are made from either stainless steel or cast iron. It is best to avoid aluminum and nonstick cookware, as the aluminum enters your food and can be toxic, and the nonstick surface may flake and also be absorbed into your food. For baking, stainless steel, glass, and earthenware are the most beneficial.

One more important thing to consider is your heat source. Gas stoves and ovens are highly recommended over electric and microwave. The gas flame affords greater control in cooking, and the safety of microwave cooking is questionable.

SUGGESTED COOKING EQUIPMENT

Pots and Pans

- Stainless-steel pressure cooker
- 9-inch cast-iron pan with a cover
- 3-quart stainless-steel soup pot with cover
- 2-quart stainless-steel saucepan with cover
- 1-quart stainless-steel saucepan with cover
- Large stainless-steel frying pan

Bakeware

- Stainless-steel 9- x 13-inch cookie sheet
- Stainless-steel or glass loaf pan
- Glass 9- x 13-inch lasagna pan
- Glass or stainless-steel 9-inch pie plate
- 8- or 9-inch stainless-steel round layer pan *or*
- 8- or 9-inch square glass or stainless-steel baking dish

Bowls and Extras

- Set of stainless-steel or glass mixing bowls
- Large strainer
- Tightly meshed strainer (for washing sesame seeds)
- 10-inch suribachi (a bowl with ridges inside used for grinding)
- 12-inch surikogi (pestle)
  (I recommend the large surikogi so it can be used as a rolling pin.)
- Stainless-steel vegetable steamer
- Bamboo steamer (can be used for reheating by placing your food on a plate and putting the plate in the steamer—almost as fast as a microwave oven but much safer)
- Glass teapot
- Deep-fry basket
  I use this item for boiling—place your food in the basket, lower it into the boiling water, and lift out when done. No more fishing around the boiling water for that last piece of cabbage, or pouring the water and food into another bowl with a strainer inside it, and then pouring the cooking water back into the pot to be boiled again. This idea was suggested by a friend and teacher of mine, Bonnie Breidenbach, who is from Michigan.
- Stainless-steel food mill
- Vegetable press
- Wooden cutting board

Other Utensils

- Ginger grater
- Larger grater
- 3 wooden mixing spoons
- Set of large chopsticks for cooking
- Stainless-steel spatula
- Rubber spatula
- Whisk
- Set of measuring spoons
- Set of measuring cups
- Potato masher
- 1 or 2 flame deflectors

- Good-quality vegetable cutting knife with wide blade
- Paring knife
- Several bamboo sushi mats for making sushi and for covering bowls of food

Electric Items (not essential, but useful)

- Food processor or blender
- Toaster oven

SUGGESTED LIST OF STAPLE FOODS

This is a basic list of food suggestions and is by no means inexhaustible.

- Grains: brown rice (short and medium grain), millet, bulghur wheat, sweet rice, rolled oats, barley, couscous, and rice cakes.
- Beans: azukis, lentils, chickpeas, and pinto beans.
- Flour Products: whole-wheat and whole-wheat pastry flours, sourdough rye or whole-wheat bread without yeast, cornmeal, whole-grain crackers, soba noodles, somen noodles, lasagna noodles (whole wheat or artichoke), and udon noodles.
- Sea Vegetables: kombu, wakame, hiziki and/or arame, agar-agar, and nori.
- Dried Fruits, Nuts, and Seeds: raisins, apricots, sesame seeds, sunflower seeds, pumpkin seeds, almonds, pecans, walnuts, and chestnuts.
- Condiments and Herbs: miso, kuzu, brown rice vinegar, tamari, fresh ginger, natural prepared mustard, umeboshi plums, umeboshi vinegar, garlic, dry mustard, and others herbs as needed.
- Beverages: bancha tea, grain coffee, barley tea, apple juice or cider, sparkling water, spring water, nonalcoholic beer (a nice treat once in a while), and sake.
- Fresh Fruit: variety of seasonal fruit.
  I would include lemons here, as I use them regularly. Because they have healing properties and can be used in relatively small amounts compared to other fruits, I feel that lemons are complementary and beneficial to the macrobiotic diet.
- Fresh Vegetables: variety of seasonal vegetables, including root vegetables, ground vegetables, and leafy vegetables.
- Oils: light sesame (dark sesame and olive need no refrigeration), corn oil, peanut butter or sesame butter, and tahini.

- Sweets: barley malt, rice syrup, maple syrup, apple butter, amasake, and unsweetened natural applesauce.
- Others: tofu, tempeh, mochi, sauerkraut, and dill pickles.

LEFTOVERS

Leftover grain, bean, and vegetable dishes are often just the keys you need to unlock your hidden creativity. Leftover grains and beans, with the addition of a small amount of flour and seasonings, can become pan-fried burgers served on whole-grain sourdough bread with mustard, sauerkraut, and grilled onions. Or they can be transformed into vegetable "meatballs" smothered in a rich vegetable sauce and served over rice. Some of your favorite soups may simply be a concoction of leftovers with the addition of a little of this or that. Lightly steamed leftover vegetables can be added to freshly steamed ones, tossed with an oil and umeboshi vinegar dressing, and served an hour or two later as a marinated vegetable salad. Cooked noodles or whole grains can be pan-fried in a small amount of oil with vegetables, beans, tofu, tempeh, or seitan for a complete "meal-in-one-pan." From bean salads to spreads, sautéed grains to croquettes, and plain vegetable dishes to creamy soups, leftovers only need a little bit of love, creativity, and appetite to be transformed into wonderful recipes that can become standards in your kitchen.

A BALANCED MEAL

People often wonder what constitutes a complete macrobiotic meal. An evening meal may be organized as follows: appetizer; soup; grain; long-cooked vegetable; short-cooked vegetable or salad; bean, bean product, seitan, or fish; sea vegetable; pickle; dessert; and tea. This may seem like a great deal to eat at one meal, but it is a general outline. The appetizer and dessert are optional. Other food categories may be combined, such as a bean and vegetable stew prepared with a piece of kombu seaweed. That would combine your bean, long-cooked vegetable, and sea vegetable.

This is only a basic meal plan. It is not meant to convey that all macrobiotic people must prepare and eat a ten-dish meal every night. But it does give an idea of what a balanced meal is all about—something cooked a long time balanced with something cooked a short time or not cooked at all; something more plain balanced with something more seasoned; or a light, liquidy food balanced with a more dense, concentrated food.

The attempt to prepare a balanced meal takes the following into consideration:

- The physical makeup of the foods themselves.
- The textures of foods.
- The five tastes—pungent, sweet, sour, salty, bitter.
- The colors of foods.
- The time of year the meal is being prepared.
- The person(s) who will be eating the meal.
- The energetic qualities of the various foods within the meal.

This may sound extremely complicated, but many people unconsciously incorporate these aspects of food preparation into their daily routine. They may serve something bland with something spicy, a light food in hot weather, and white spaghetti with red sauce, a green salad, and tan-colored bread.

Because many of the foods included in whole-foods cookery may be unfamiliar, it is important to realize how to balance these foods to achieve your greatest health potential. After a short while, the notion of a "balanced meal" may come naturally.

Meal presentation is almost as important as the food itself. A very plain meal will be much more appetizing if presented in an attractive way. A meal that is pleasing to the eye and garnished with color in mind may even taste better than the same exact meal presented in a careless manner.

EATING OUT

Now that you know what macrobiotics is all about, and your kitchen is stocked and your recipes organized, you may find that, as much as you love to cook, there are some days when you just don't feel like it. Or, you may decide to travel to a place where kitchen facilities won't be available. At these times, it is helpful to have an idea of where to eat good-quality, wholesome food. Unless you are traveling in a foreign country or to a very small town, some or all of these restaurant ideas will be available.

In macrobiotic restaurants, order freely unless you are on a restricted macrobiotic diet. Natural foods restaurants often serve one or two macrobiotic platters. Their casseroles, soups, and main dishes are usually carefully prepared and delicious. However, if a dairy-free diet is your preference, watch out for dairy products hidden in soups, salad dressings, main dishes, and desserts. Ask questions!

Mexican restaurants offer bean tacos, bean burritos, rice, salad, guacamole, and steamed tortillas that make a hearty meal for lunch or dinner. Before ordering, ask if lard is used in the cooking. Many Mexican restaurants use lard in their beans and fried foods.

Chinese restaurants all serve rice, noodles, and an assortment of vegetables. Lard is usually used in their deep-fried foods, while peanut oil is used in their stir-fried dishes. Ask to have your food prepared without MSG (monosodium glutamate), which is a flavor enhancer that can cause excessive thirst and other more extreme symptoms in sensitive individuals. Avoid sweet-and-sour dishes and sauces, as they are loaded with sugar.

Japanese restaurants offer an assortment of interesting grain, vegetable, and fish dishes usually presented in an artistic fashion. Many Japanese restaurants use a great deal of sugar, even in their vegetables and sushi. It may not be possible to avoid eating sugar in this situation. Ask if your food can be prepared without MSG. The miso soup is often prepared with chicken broth instead of water or vegetable stock.

Middle Eastern restaurants serve a variety of vegetable-quality dishes such as hummus, tabouli salad, rice-stuffed grape leaves, falafels, lentil soup, various vegetables, and rice. Though the food is well seasoned and delicious, it is oily. If you are on an oil-restricted diet or simply choose not to eat much oil, then another type of restaurant would be a wiser choice.

Italian restaurants are great for satisfying a pasta craving, aside from cravings for other well-known favorites. Linguine with white clam sauce, salad, vegetables (hold the butter and Parmesan cheese, please), pasta sautéed with vegetables, and mushroom, onion, and green-pepper pizza without cheese (a special order), are all served. Many fine Italian restaurants also serve a variety of fresh seafood.

Seafood restaurants serve fish and seafood that is usually prepared in a variety of ways—baked, broiled, in salads, and deep-fried. Since most restaurants bake or broil their fish with butter, you may have to request that no butter be used in the preparation of your dish.

Wherever you decide to eat, enjoy and appreciate your food, the service, and the atmosphere. Have a good time!

1.

❈   ❈   ❈

Breakfast

Vegetables for breakfast! The macrobiotic diet sometimes includes vegetables and rice for breakfast, but there is no steadfast rule to that effect. Grains, in some form, are usually served because they gradually raise your blood sugar, which is low after fasting overnight, and help sustain the energy needed to perform your morning activities.

Breakfast is usually a fairly simple meal, not too spicy or salty. A morning meal that is spicy or salty may make you want to drink liquids and eat sweets all day.

Like any other meal, breakfast is meant to be enjoyed. Whether or not you choose to eat vegetables, try to enjoy and appreciate the day's first meal, and set a peaceful, relaxed tone for the rest of the day.

Ramen Pancake with Tofu Cream Dressing

YIELD: 2 SERVINGS

Pancake
1½ cups water
1 package Ramen
1–2 teaspoons Ramen seasoning
1 tablespoon light sesame oil

Tofu Cream Dressing
¼ pound tofu
1 umeboshi plum, pitted
Pinch sea salt
1 tablespoon olive oil
6–8 tablespoons water
1 teaspoon rice vinegar

Garnish
2 scallions, sliced

Boil 1½ cups water in medium-sized saucepan. Add Ramen, lower heat, and simmer for 5 minutes. Add 1 teaspoon of Ramen seasoning, cover saucepan, and set aside for at least 20 minutes. Liquid and seasonings will absorb into noodles.

While noodles are resting, boil tofu for 1 minute, drain, and place in blender or food processor with remaining dressing ingredients. Purée until creamy.

Heat sesame oil over medium heat in a 9-inch or larger skillet (big enough to hold all the noodles). Noodles will now be molded to size of original saucepan. Lift them from saucepan with spatula, trying to maintain their shape. Add molded, noodle pancake to hot oil. Pan-fry for 5 minutes, turn over with spatula, and pan-fry for another 5 minutes. Serve hot, topped with tofu cream dressing and sliced scallions.

Mochi Sandwiches

YIELD: 4–6 SERVINGS

2 packages plain mochi

CHOOSE ONE OF THE FOLLOWING FILLINGS:

Broiled Tofu Filling
1 pound tofu
1–2 tablespoons tamari
1–2 teaspoons grated ginger

Dried Fruit Filling
¼ cup dried apricots
¼ cup prunes, pitted
1 cup toasted sunflower seeds (See page 30 for seed-toasting directions.)

Nut or Seed Butter
almond, cashew, peanut, or sesame butter

Fruit Spread
apple, raspberry, strawberry, or blueberry

Maple Butter
maple butter

Grain-Sweetened Chocolate Chips
grain-sweetened chocolate chips placed in the pocket of hot mochi
Nuts or nut butter (optional)

Slice each package of mochi into 6 sections, each about 2 inches square. Bake mochi pieces on lightly oiled baking sheet for 15–20 minutes at 400°F, or until they are puffed and crispy on the outside. Make a slit on one side of each piece of mochi and fill with either broiled tofu or dried fruit filling.

To prepare broiled tofu, slice tofu block into ¼-inch-thick slices and transfer to unoiled 9- × 13-inch baking sheet. Sprinkle each slice with a few drops of tamari and some grated ginger. Broil for 5 minutes and serve one slice of tofu inside each piece of mochi.

To prepare dried fruit, soak apricots and prunes in water to cover overnight. Place a piece of soaked fruit and a teaspoon of sunflower seeds inside each piece of mochi.

Variety Soft Rice

YIELD: 2–3 SERVINGS

Basic Rice
1 cup brown rice
5 cups water
⅛ teaspoon sea salt

Variety of Toppings
Toasted peanuts (See page 30 for nut-toasting directions.)
Crispy Brown Rice (Can be found at your natural foods store.)
Toasted sunflower seeds (See page 30 for seed-toasting directions.)
Raisins
Barley malt
Toasted sesame seeds (See page 30 for seed-toasting directions.)

Pressure-cook rice, water, and sea salt for 50 minutes. (For boiling directions, please refer to Basic Grain Cooking Chart on page 50.) Serve with a variety of toppings.

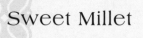

Apricot Soft Rice

YIELD 2–3 SERVINGS

1 cup short-grain brown rice
⅛ teaspoon sea salt
5 cups water
½ cup dried apricots

Pressure-cook all ingredients for 50 minutes. (If boiling directions are needed, please refer to Basic Grain Cooking Chart on page 50.) Serve hot, topped with nuts or seeds if desired.

Sweet Millet

YIELD: 4 SERVINGS

Pudding
1 cup raisin juice
3 cups water
1 cup uncooked millet
⅛ teaspoon sea salt
4 medium carrots, peeled and sliced

Sauce
Soaked raisins, left over from pudding recipe
1 tablespoon kuzu, dissolved in 1 cup water
Pinch sea salt
2 tablespoons barley malt
½ teaspoon vanilla
½ cup toasted walnuts (See page 30 for nut-toasting directions.)

To make raisin juice, bring 1 cup of raisins to boil in 2 cups of water. Lower heat, and simmer for about 15 minutes. Pour raisins and liquid through a strainer placed in a bowl. Reserve raisins for sauce and use liquid in cooking millet.

Bring millet, raisin juice, 1 cup water, sea salt, and carrots to boil in a medium-sized saucepan. Lower heat, cover, and simmer for 30 minutes. Purée hot millet mixture in a food mill, and set aside.

To prepare sauce, combine soaked raisins, dissolved kuzu, sea salt, barley malt, vanilla, and walnuts in small saucepan. Stir over medium heat until sauce thickens—about 5 minutes. Serve warm sauce over each serving of millet pudding.

Apple Granola

YIELD: ABOUT 3 CUPS

2 cups uncooked rolled oats
1 cup almonds, sunflower seeds, walnuts, pecans, or cashews; chopped
⅓ cup apple concentrate
¼ cup light sesame oil
¼ teaspoon sea salt
½ teaspoon vanilla

Combine ingredients, mixing well. Spread on a 9- × 13-inch cookie sheet and bake at 350°F for about 2 minutes, until golden brown. After 15 minutes, stir granola mixture, and return to oven for 5 more minutes. Cool, then store in tightly covered container.

Variations

- Add ¼ cup shredded coconut to oat mixture before baking.
- Add ½ cup raisins or chopped dates to granola after it has been baked.

Scrambled Tofu

YIELD: 4 SERVINGS

> *1 medium onion, diced*
> *1 teaspoon light or dark sesame oil*
> *8 medium mushrooms, sliced*
> **½ green or red pepper, diced*
> *¼ teaspoon sea salt*
> *1 pound tofu*
> *¼ teaspoon turmeric*

Sauté onion in oil in a medium-sized frying pan. Add mushrooms, green or red pepper, and sea salt. Sauté until pepper is tender. Add tofu, mashing it with a wooden spoon to break it into small pieces. Continue to sauté for 5–8 more minutes, stirring in turmeric as it cooks. Serve tofu hot with toast, muffins, mochi, or rice cakes.

Scrambled Tofu Satori

by Satori Natural Foods Restaurant

YIELD: 6–8 SERVINGS

> *2 cloves garlic*
> *½ teaspoon grated ginger*
> *3 teaspoons sesame or olive oil*
> *1 medium onion*

---

*Not recommended on a strict macrobiotic diet.

*1 medium green pepper
1 medium carrot, peeled
Pinch sea salt
3 pounds tofu
¼ teaspoon turmeric
Tamari or sea salt to taste

Sauté garlic and ginger in a lightly oiled skillet. Dice onion, green pepper, and carrot and add to hot skillet. Add pinch of sea salt and sauté until soft. Mash the 3 squares of drained tofu into skillet, using fork or potato masher. Cook on high flame for 5–7 minutes. Add turmeric for a yellow color. Add sea salt or tamari to taste.

Carrot-Couscous Muffins

YIELD: 6 MUFFINS

1½ large carrots, peeled and thinly sliced
¼ cup amasake
½ cup raisins
3 cups water
1½ cups uncooked couscous
¼ teaspoon sea salt
¼ teaspoon cardamom, coriander, or cinnamon

Bring carrots, amasake, raisins, and water to boil in a medium-sized saucepan. Lower heat, cover, and simmer until carrots are very soft—about 15 minutes. Remove carrots and raisins with slotted spoon or mesh strainer, purée through a food mill, and set aside.

Add couscous, sea salt, and spices to the hot liquid left in pan. Bring to boil, lower heat, and simmer for about 10 minutes, until all the liquid is absorbed.

---

*Not recommended on a strict macrobiotic diet.

Combine puréed carrot mixture with couscous and spoon into muffin cups. Cool thoroughly. Run a knife around the edge of each muffin, unmold, and serve.

Variations

- Add ¼ cup chopped nuts or seeds to cooked couscous mixture before pressing it into muffin cups.
- Use barley malt in place of amasake.
- Use 1½ large parsnips, peeled and thinly sliced, or 1 small squash, peeled and thinly sliced, in place of carrots.

Raisin-Walnut Muffins

by Charles Gary and Mary David

YIELD: 6–8 MUFFINS

½ cup raisins
1½ cups whole-wheat pastry flour
½ cup sweet rice flour
¼ teaspoon sea salt
¼ cup corn oil
1 tablespoon kuzu
¼ cup cool water
1 cup chopped walnuts
1 cup apple juice

Boil raisins in water to cover for 10 minutes. Combine flours and salt in large mixing bowl. Rub corn oil into flour mixture with your hands.

Dissolve kuzu into ¼ cup cool water and stir it into boiling raisins until thick. Remove from heat and cool slightly. Stir raisins, nuts, and apple juice into flour mixture to form a thick, but pourable, batter. Adjust amount of apple juice if necessary.

Pour into oiled muffin tin and bake at 400°F for about 30 minutes until golden brown and springy to touch.

Blueberry Muffins

by Muriel Crisara

YIELD: 6 MUFFINS

> *2 cups whole-wheat pastry flour*
> *1 teaspoon baking powder*
> *1 teaspoon baking soda*
> *1 teaspoon sea salt*
> *2 eggs*
> *¼ cup canola oil*
> *½ cup honey*
> *8 ounces soy milk*
> *1 cup blueberries*
> *½ cup chopped nuts (optional)*

Blend flour, baking powder, baking soda, and sea salt in a mixing bowl and set aside. In another mixing bowl, add eggs, oil, honey, and soy milk and beat together. Add mixture to dry ingredients and mix together well. Stir in blueberries and nuts. Distribute batter evenly among 6 oiled muffin cups. Bake at 350°F for 18–20 minutes. Let cool slightly and run a knife around each muffin before removing.

Rice and Onion Muffins

YIELD: 6 SMALL MUFFINS

> *2 cups cooked rice (pressed into measuring container)*
> *1¼ cups whole-wheat pastry flour*
> *½ cup diced onion*

2 tablespoons toasted poppy seeds (See page 30 for seed-toasting directions.)
½ teaspoon sea salt
2 tablespoons light sesame oil
1 teaspoon baking powder
1½ cups water

Gently stir all ingredients together in a medium-sized mixing bowl. Oil 6 muffin cups. Fill each one halfway, and bake at 350°F for about 30 minutes. Let cool slightly and run a knife around each muffin before removing.

Cinnamon Muffins

YIELD: 6 SMALL MUFFINS

2 cups whole-wheat pastry flour
1 tablespoon baking powder
½ teaspoon sea salt
2 tablespoons light sesame oil
1¾ cups water
1 tablespoon rice syrup
¼ cup raisins
½ teaspoon cinnamon

Combine flour, baking powder, and sea salt in medium-sized mixing bowl. Stir in oil, water, rice syrup, raisins, and cinnamon. Distribute batter evenly among 6 oiled muffin cups. Bake at 350°F for about 30 minutes. Let muffins cool and run a knife around the edge of each one before removing.

Seed- and Nut-Toasting Directions

Poppy seeds: Put seeds in a pan over medium heat. Stir for about 5 minutes, until they are fragrant.

Sunflower seeds: Put seeds in a pan over medium heat. Slowly stir with a wooden spoon until the seeds are lightly toasted.

Sesame seeds: First, rinse the seeds in a fine-mesh strainer, removing any stones or sticks. Dry-roast in a frying pan or saucepan until the seeds pop and are fragrant.

Nuts: Place on a baking pan in a 350°F oven for 10 to 15 minutes, until nuts are fragrant and a light golden brown on the inside.

Sunflower Buckwheat Muffins

YIELD: 10 SMALL MUFFINS

2 cups uncooked buckwheat groats
¼ teaspoon sea salt
1 cup apple juice
3 cups water
2 tablespoons raisins
1 teaspoon coriander
¼ cup sunflower seeds (See above for seed-toasting directions.)
1 tablespoon toasted sesame seeds (See above for seed-toasting directions.)

Bring buckwheat, sea salt, apple juice, water, raisins, and coriander to boil in a medium-sized saucepan. Lower heat, cover, and simmer for about 20 minutes or until all the liquid has been absorbed. Stir seeds into cooked buckwheat mixture. Spoon mixture into muffin cups, and cool. Run a knife around the edge of each muffin and remove by turning upside down onto a plate. Serve as a snack or with a meal.

2.

Soup

Whether it be a bowl of steaming hot soup on a chilly night, or a bowl of cold soup on a hot summer afternoon, soups add a special touch to any meal. The macrobiotic diet recommends one to two bowls of soup every day. Soup helps prepare your digestion for the remainder of your meal. It slows you down, and often has a soothing, calming effect on your body after a hectic day.

Soups can be prepared from almost any of the foods suggested on the standard macrobiotic diet. Culinary delights may be created by using your time, energy, imagination, and taste buds in order to create an interesting soup that may prove to make any meal a special one.

Christina Pirello

At age twenty-six, after being diagnosed with terminal leukemia, Christina Pirello turned to a nutritional approach—whole foods—to cure herself. Since then, her passion and commitment to whole foods has grown over the last sixteen years as she has taught whole-foods cooking classes and conducted lifestyle seminars and lectures on the power of food in our lives.

Since 1989, she and her husband have been publishing a bimonthly whole-foods magazine, *Christina Cooks* and operating Christina Trips, a travel company that specializes in healthy vacations to exotic destinations. She is the Emmy Award–winning host of the PBS series *Christina Cooks* and is the author of the best-selling cookbook *Cooking the Whole Foods Way,* as well as *Cook Your Way to the Life You Want, Glow: A Prescription for Radiant Health and Beauty,* and *Christina Cooks: Everything You've Ever Wanted to Know About Natural Foods, but Were Afraid to Ask.*

Christina believes there's nothing quite as beautifying as sweet, creamy soups. The smooth, creamy consistency of her Sweet Parsnip Soup with Hazelnut Pesto is a fountain of youth that helps to strengthen the blood to nourish our skin.

Sweet Parsnip Soup with Hazelnut Pesto

by Christina Pirello
author of *Glow: A Prescription for Radiant Health and Beauty*

YIELD: 6–8 SERVINGS

1 onion, diced
1 small leek, split lengthwise, rinsed well, diced
6 parsnips, peeled and diced
1 small butternut squash, halved, seeded, diced
3 cups plain soy milk or rice milk
3 cups spring or filtered water

¼ cup mirin
2½ teaspoons white miso
Small bunch fresh parsley, minced for garnish

Hazelnut Pesto
1 cup hazelnuts, oven toasted, skinned
1 cup loosely packed fresh basil leaves
1 cup loosely packed fresh Italian flat-leaf parsley leaves
3 shallots, diced
¾ cup extra-virgin olive oil
2 teaspoons white miso
2 teaspoons umeboshi vinegar or fresh lemon juice
1 teaspoon brown rice syrup

Layer vegetables in a soup pot in the order listed. Gently add rice or soy milk, water, and mirin. Cover and bring to a boil over medium heat. Reduce heat to low and simmer until parsnips and squash are quite soft, about 30 minutes. Remove a small amount of broth, dissolve miso and stir into soup. Simmer, uncovered for 3–4 minutes to activate enzyme activity.

While the soup cooks, make the pesto. Combine all ingredients in a food processor and purée until smooth. You will have more pesto than you may need for this recipe. It will keep, refrigerated, for about a week.

Transfer soup, by ladles, through a chinois or food mill, to create a smooth purée. Return to pot and simmer for 1 minute. Serve, garnished with a generous dollop of pesto and sprinkled with minced parsley.

NOTE: To roast hazelnuts, arrange nuts on a baking sheet and bake at 325° for about 15–20 minutes, until fragrant. Transfer nuts to a paper bag and allow skins to loosen in the steam for about 10 minutes. Then rub nuts in a towel to remove the skins.

Cream of Broccoli Soup

YIELD: 4 SERVINGS

1 medium onion, chopped
1 teaspoon dark sesame oil
3 cups water
4 cups chopped broccoli
1 medium parsnip, peeled and diced
1 tablespoon rice flour
1 teaspoon sea salt
1 cup plain soy milk
Chopped scallions and croutons to garnish

Sauté onion in oil until transparent in a medium-sized saucepan. Add water, chopped broccoli, parsnip, and sea salt. Bring to boil, lower heat and simmer for about 15 minutes or until the broccoli and parsnips are soft. Put rice flour and sea salt in a blender or food processor and purée. Add 1 cup of plain soy milk to the soup and continue to simmer until ready to serve. Garnish with chopped scallions and croutons.

Miso Corn Soup

YIELD: 4 SERVINGS

1 piece wakame, 4 inches long
4 cups water
¾ cup peas
½ medium carrot, peeled and cut into rounds
⅛ teaspoon garlic powder
2 ears corn
2–3 teaspoons light miso

Soak wakame in water to cover for 5–10 minutes, or until soft. Slice out stems and discard, or reserve them to cook with a grain. Thinly slice leafy portion of wakame and combine it with water, peas, carrot rounds, and garlic powder in a 2-quart or larger saucepan. Cut corn off cobs and add to soup. Bring soup to boil, lower heat, and simmer for 20 minutes. Transfer a few tablespoons of soup broth to a small bowl and purée miso and broth together with a spoon or small whisk. Add miso purée to soup and simmer for 3–5 minutes before serving.

Muriel Crisara

Muriel Crisara, a longtime practitioner of the macrobiotic way of life and former owner of the Sprout House, a macrobiotic store in Grosse Point, Michigan, is now a retired macrobiotic consultant on Cape Cod. Because of her knowledge and enthusiasm for everything macrobiotic, people continue to seek her out for cooking classes and answers to questions about macrobiotic philosophy.

Muriel's recipes for squash soup and Alfredo sauce include Herbamare, an organic seasoning blend that includes sea salt, celery stalk, celery leaves, leeks, watercress, garden cress, onions, chives, parsley, lovage, garlic, basil, marjoram, rosemary, thyme, and kelp.

Squash Soup

YIELD: 2–3 SERVINGS

1 medium butternut squash
1 cup water
3 cloves garlic
Herbamare
½ cup plain soy milk (optional)

Cut squash into halves and place facedown on baking pan. Pour 1 cup of water over squash. Place garlic cloves with their peels still on onto a separate cooking sheet or baking dish. Bake all at 350°F until squash is tender, 45 minutes to 1 hour depending on the size of the squash.* Scoop squash out of peels and put in blender. Remove garlic cloves from their peels and add to blender. Blend for a few minutes on a medium speed until it reaches a creamy consistency. This will make a very thick soup. Add soy milk if the soup appears to be too thick to blend thoroughly or if you desire a thinner mixture. Add Herbamare to taste. Serve hot.

Sunchoke Vegetable Soup

YIELD: 4 SERVINGS

1 piece wakame, 6 inches long
4 cups water or vegetable stock
3 sunchokes (also called Jerusalem artichokes), sliced
1 large onion, sliced
1 medium carrot, peeled and sliced
3 shiitake mushrooms, soaked in ¼ cup water for 10 minutes, and sliced
½ teaspoon dill
½ teaspoon ground bay leaf
1 cup fresh peas
1 tablespoon barley miso

Soak wakame in water to cover for about 10 minutes or until soft. Remove from water and cut into small pieces, removing stem. The stem may be chopped and added to your next pot of grains or beans, or discarded.

Combine wakame, water or stock, sunchokes, onion, carrot, shiitake mushrooms, dill, and bay leaf in a 2-quart or larger saucepan. Bring vegetable mixture to boil, lower heat, and simmer for 35 minutes. Add peas and simmer for about 10 more minutes.

---

*Check squash periodically, adding ¼ cup water if the pan is dry. This will prevent the squash from burning and giving the soup a bitter taste.

Remove a small amount of soup broth and purée it with the miso in a blender, food mill, or food processor. Add miso purée to soup. Simmer for another 3–5 minutes. Do not boil once miso has been added, as this destroys miso's valuable digestive enzymes. Serve hot.

Chilled Carrot-Beet Soup

YIELD: 4 SERVINGS

1 large or 2 small cloves garlic, minced
1 medium onion, sliced
1 teaspoon olive oil
5 large carrots, peeled and sliced
1 medium beet, peeled and sliced
¼ teaspoon basil
2 teaspoons umeboshi plum paste
2½ cups water
1 teaspoon dark miso
*1 tablespoon lemon juice

Topping
1 recipe tofu cream dressing (See recipe on page 20 or use a
commercially prepared soy or tofu sour cream.)

Sauté garlic and onion in oil in a 4-quart or larger pressure cooker for a few minutes. Add carrots, beet, basil, umeboshi plum paste, and water. Pressure-cook for 20 minutes. If boiling, follow the same procedure as above, but instead of pressure-cooking, bring ingredients to boil, lower heat, and simmer until vegetables are very soft.

Purée the hot, cooked vegetables in a food mill or blender and return purée to pot. Add miso and simmer soup for 3–5 minutes. Stir in lemon juice and chill.

Prepare tofu cream and serve each portion of soup topped with a heaping tablespoon of tofu cream.

---

*Not recommended on a strict macrobiotic diet.

Navy Bean Soup

Yield: 4 servings

1 piece of cheesecloth, 4 inches square
1 celery stalk, cut in chunks
1 small sprig parsley
*½ lemon
1 bay leaf
1 piece of cotton string
1 cup uncooked navy beans
4 cups water
1 piece kombu, 4 inches long
1 medium onion, thinly sliced
3 medium carrots, peeled and sliced
1 cup sliced green beans
1–2 tablespoons tamari or 1 tablespoon dark miso
2 scallions, sliced

Make a cheesecloth pouch containing celery, parsley, lemon, and bay leaf. Tie pouch closed with cotton string. Pressure-cook navy beans, water, kombu, onion, carrots, green beans, and cheesecloth pouch for 50 minutes. Beans should become very soft.

After opening pressure cooker, squeeze cheesecloth pouch into broth and remove it from cooked bean mixture. Remove and dice kombu and return it to soup.

If using tamari, add it to hot soup broth. If using miso, spoon some hot soup broth into a small bowl, add miso, and purée before adding miso to soup. In either case, simmer soup for 3–5 minutes before serving. Garnish with sliced scallions, and serve.

---

*Not recommended on a strict macrobiotic diet.

Kidney Bean–Seitan Chili

YIELD: 4 SERVINGS

Basic Beans
1½ cups uncooked kidney beans
4 cups water
1 bay leaf
1 piece kombu, 3 inches long

Seitan
2 cups whole wheat flour
1 cup water

Seitan Broth
2 cups water
1 tablespoon tamari

Vegetables and Seasonings
2 gloves garlic, minced
1 medium onion, chopped
*1 green pepper, chopped
½ teaspoon ground cumin
½–¾ teaspoon sea salt
1 teaspoon cayenne pepper
1 teaspoon corn oil

Pressure-cook kidney beans, water, bay leaf, and kombu for 1 hour or until beans are soft. (If boiling, please refer to Basic Bean Cooking Chart on page 98 for directions.)

While beans are cooking, prepare seitan as in the Seitan Wellington recipe on pages

---

*Not recommended on a strict macrobiotic diet.

92–93, using 2 cups whole-wheat flour and 1 cup of water. Tear uncooked seitan into small pieces, about ½-inch long and ¼-inch wide. Combine water, kombu, tamari, and seitan pieces in medium-sized saucepan and simmer for 30 minutes. Do not boil or seitan will become spongy.

Sauté garlic, onion, green pepper, cumin, sea salt, and cayenne pepper in corn oil for 5 minutes or until green pepper is tender. Set aside.

Remove seitan from broth with slotted spoon and transfer it to cooked kidney beans in pressure cooker. Stir sautéed vegetables into kidney-bean mixture. Stir over low heat for a few minutes to allow flavors to blend. Add some seitan broth to the chili if it appears to be too thick. If not, reserve seitan broth to be used as soup stock.

Serve chili hot, garnished with croutons or chopped scallions, if desired.

Lentil Soup

Yield: 4 servings

1 cup uncooked lentils
3 cups water
1 piece kombu, 4 inches long
1 bay leaf
1 medium onion, sliced
½ teaspoon olive oil
2 celery stalks, sliced
2 medium turnips, peeled and sliced
¼ cup chopped parsley
1 tablespoon miso
*Lemon slices

Pressure-cook lentils with water, kombu, and bay leaf for 30 minutes. (If boiling is preferred, see Basic Bean Cooking Chart on page 98 for instructions.) Sauté onion in oil until it is transparent. Add celery and turnips and cook until vegetables are tender.

---

*Not recommended on a strict macrobiotic diet.

When lentils are cooked, remove bay leaf and kombu. Discard bay leaf, slice kombu, and return kombu to pot. Add sautéed vegetables and parsley to lentil mixture. Adjust the amount of water in the soup, if necessary.

Purée miso with a spoon or small whisk in a small bowl with ¼ cup of soup broth. Add miso purée to soup and simmer for a few more minutes. Serve hot, garnished with lemon slices if desired.

Purple Passion Stew

by Jessica Porter

YIELD: 4 SERVINGS

> *1 piece of kombu, 2 inches long*
> *1 medium daikon, sliced*
> *½ small red cabbage or ¼ large red cabbage, chopped*
> *1 cup water*
> *1 tablespoon umeboshi vinegar*

Soak kombu for several minutes (usually 5–7) until soft enough to cut. Slice kombu into thin strips and place in the bottom of a heavy, 2-quart pot. Slice daikon into one-inch rounds and add to pot. Chop cabbage into bite-sized pieces and place on top. Pour 1 cup water into the pot (or enough to measure about 1 inch in the pot). Add umeboshi vinegar. Cover and bring to a boil. Reduce flame to low and simmer for 30 minutes. Remove from heat and stir so that the daikon gets stained purple. Serve hot.

Jessica Porter

Portland, Maine

After being trained in macrobiotics at the Kushi Institute, Jessica Porter served for two years as the manager of the Institute's Way of Health program for seriously ill people looking to improve their health through macrobiotics. She then took her rich experience in macrobiotic cooking, philosophy, and health on the road as traveling chef for private clients. Currently, Jessica teaches cooking classes at the Five Seasons Whole Food Cooking School in Portland, Maine, and is the author of an upcoming pop culture guide to the macrobiotic way of life.

   Her recipe for Purple Passion stew, while technically not a stew, is a variation on nishime-style cooking. Its bright purple color and slightly sour taste make for a bold, exotic character on the plate. This particular hue, almost a fuchsia, is a great complement to the bright greens and oranges of other vegetables.

Middle Eastern Chickpea Soup

YIELD: 4 SERVINGS

2 cups uncooked chickpeas
1 piece kombu, 4 inches long
1 bay leaf
7 cups water
2 cloves garlic, minced
⅛ teaspoon sea salt
2 teaspoons light miso
*1 lemon, sliced

---

*Not recommended on a strict macrobiotic diet.

Pressure-cook chickpeas, kombu, bay leaf, and water in a 4-quart or larger pressure cooker for 2 hours or until chickpeas are very soft. (If boiling, please refer to Basic Bean Cooking Chart on page 98 for directions.) Purée cooked chickpeas, kombu, garlic, sea salt, and miso in a food mill or blender—remove bay leaf before puréeing and discard. Transfer soup back to pressure cooker or pot and simmer for about 5 minutes before serving. Add one slice of lemon to each bowl of soup if desired.

Pinto Bean–Red Pepper Soup

YIELD: 4 SERVINGS

1 cup uncooked pinto beans
4 cups water
1 piece kombu, 6 inches long, cut or broken into small pieces
1 bay leaf
*1 red bell pepper, chopped
1 celery stalk, sliced
½ cup uncooked artichoke or whole-wheat shells, macaroni, or rotini
1½ tablespoons tamari

Pressure-cook pinto beans, water, kombu, bay leaf, red pepper, and celery for 60 minutes. (If boiling, please refer to Basic Bean Cooking Chart on page 98 for directions.) While bean mixture is cooking, boil shells, macaroni, or rotini for 10 minutes or until tender. Set aside. Stir tamari and cooked pasta into cooked beans. Add more water to thin soup, if desired. Simmer for 3–5 minutes and serve hot.

---

*Not recommended on a strict macrobiotic diet.

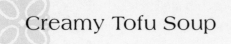

Creamy Tofu Soup

YIELD: 4 SERVINGS

> ½ pound tofu
> 3 celery stalks, diced
> 1 medium onion, diced
> ½ teaspoon dark sesame oil
> 1 teaspoon sea salt
> 3 cups water
> 1 teaspoon dried dill
> 1 tablespoon whole-wheat pastry or unbleached white flour
> 1 tablespoon kuzu
> 1–2 scallions, chopped

Purée tofu in a blender with 1 cup of water and pour it into a 2-quart or larger saucepan. Sauté celery and onion in oil until onion is pearly white, adding sea salt while sautéing. Add sautéed vegetables, 3 cups water, and dill to puréed tofu. Combine flour, kuzu, and small amount of soup in a small bowl and stir until smooth. Stir kuzu mixture into soup and heat over low flame for 30 minutes, stirring often. Soup will thicken. Serve hot, garnished with chopped scallions.

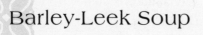

Barley-Leek Soup

YIELD: 4 SERVINGS

> 4 cups vegetable stock or water
> 1 piece kombu, 4 inches long
> 2 celery stalks, sliced

2 medium carrots, peeled and sliced
2 large leeks, sliced diagonally
¼ cup chopped parsley
2 bay leaves
¼ cup uncooked barley
1 clove garlic, minced
½ teaspoon dark sesame oil
½–1 cup more water, if needed
1 tablespoon white miso

Bring vegetable stock or water and kombu to a boil in a medium-sized saucepan. Add celery, carrots, leeks, parsley, bay leaves, and barley. Sauté garlic in oil and add to soup. Lower heat and simmer for about 1 hour. If soup becomes too thick, add ½–1 cup more water.

After 1 hour, remove bay leaves and discard. Remove kombu, slice, and return it to soup. Purée miso with a spoon or small whisk in a small bowl with ¼ cup water. Add miso purée to soup and simmer a few more minutes. Serve hot.

Variation

• Substitute millet or rice for the barley.

Broccoli-Noodle Soup

by Julia Ferre
George Ohsawa Macrobiotic Foundation

YIELD: ABOUT 10 CUPS

1 teaspoon light or dark sesame oil
1 medium onion, cut into thin crescents
1 medium bunch broccoli: stem cut in quarter rounds and flowerets cut
*   into 2-inch pieces*

8 cups boiling water
¼ teaspoon sea salt
2 cups whole-wheat ribbon noodles, lightly packed
2 tablespoons sesame butter
2–3 tablespoons soy sauce

Heat oil in heavy large-sized saucepan over medium heat. Add onions and sauté until transparent, 1 to 2 minutes. Add broccoli stems and sauté 1 minute. Add boiling water and sea salt. Cover. Bring to boil and lower heat to simmer for 10 minutes. Add noodles and broccoli flowerets. Cover and simmer for 15 minutes.

Dilute sesame butter in ¼ cup hot soup broth. Add to soup with soy sauce. Stir to heat through, but do not boil.

Julia Ferre

George Ohsawa Macrobiotic Foundation
Vega Study Center

Julia Ferre began studying macrobiotics in 1979, while attending the University of Wisconsin in Madison. She joined the Vega staff in 1981 as Cornellia Aihara's cooking assistant, and since then she has been sharing macrobiotics with others.

At the Vega Study Center, Julia taught macrobiotic classes in menu planning and cooking. She also offers cooking classes, which are designed for those who are not macrobiotic, at a local health food store.

Julia wrote a wonderful cookbook entitled *Basic Macrobiotic Cooking*.

Seitan-Noodle Soup

Yield: 4 servings

Seitan
2 cups whole-wheat flour
1 cup water

Broth
4 cups water
½ teaspoon sea salt
¼ teaspoon turmeric
¼ teaspoon thyme
1 bay leaf
1 piece kombu, 4 inches long
1 medium onion, diced

Noodles
⅛ pound uncooked somen (If noodles are held together in a bunch,
     they would measure 1 inch in diameter.)

To prepare seitan, follow the Seitan Wellington (pages 92–93) basic seitan kneading instructions, using 2 cups whole-wheat flour and 1 cup of water. Cut uncooked seitan into ½-inch cubes and set aside.

Combine broth ingredients and uncooked seitan in a 2-quart or larger saucepan. Simmer seitan mixture for 30 minutes. Do not boil, or spongy seitan will result. Remove bay leaf.

While seitan and broth are cooking, boil noodles for 7–8 minutes, drain, and set aside.

When seitan is done, add noodles, and serve hot.

Scallop Broth Over Noodles

YIELD: 3–4 SERVINGS

Broth
3½ cups water
1 teaspoon sea salt
½ pound scallops
1 small onion, diced
1 small carrot, peeled and sliced
½ teaspoon rice syrup
2 teaspoons kuzu dissolved in 2 tablespoons water

Noodles
8 ounces udon noodles

Dip for Scallops
1 tablespoon prepared mustard
1 tablespoon water
1 teaspoon mirin
1 teaspoon rice syrup

Bring water and sea salt to boil in medium-sized saucepan, add scallops, and bring to boil again. Boil for 2 minutes. Remove scallops with slotted spoon and chill until serving time.

Add onion, carrot, and rice syrup to boiling broth. Lower heat and simmer for 15 minutes until carrot slices are very soft. Transfer carrot slices to a plate, mash with a fork, and return carrot to soup. Add dissolved kuzu to broth and simmer for a few more minutes until broth becomes slightly thickened.

Boil udon noodles for about 10–12 minutes or until tender. Drain, place in bowls, and serve scallop broth over noodles.

Stir dip ingredients together and serve in a small bowl along with chilled, boiled scallops.

3.

❀ ❀ ❀

Grain

Ideally, a macrobiotic diet should consist of 50 percent grains. Because there are so many different varieties of grains, the diet is never monotonous. Grains can be made into a lightly sweetened breakfast cereal, a well-seasoned luncheon loaf, a tangy dinner salad, a flat bread, and more.

Grains are versatile, and are easy to use as a basic food choice. A variety of grains, seasonings, serving styles, and preparation techniques have been included in this chapter. Variations have also been suggested. Why not try your own variations? There are so many delicious ways to serve natural foods that it's hard to go wrong!

COOKING GRAINS

The following chart can be used as a guide for both pressure-cooking and steaming grains. Generally, all grains should be cooked with salt—a pinch of salt per cup of uncooked grain is sufficient. When grain is boiled, the grain, water, salt, and seasonings are brought to a boil. Then the heat should be lowered, and the grain should be simmered for the length of time suggested on this chart.

Basic Grain Cooking Chart		
1 cup uncooked grain	*Pressure-Cooking*	*Boiling*
Barley	1½–2 cups water for 45 minutes	2 cups water for 1 hour
Buckwheat Groats	Do not pressure-cook	1½–2 cups water for 20 minutes
Bulghur Wheat	Do not pressure-cook	1½–2 cups water for 20 minutes
Cornmeal	Do not pressure-cook	4 cups water for 30–40 minutes
Whole Dried Corn	2 cups water for 1 hour	2½–3 cups water for 3 hours or more until soft
Couscous	Do not pressure-cook	2 cups water for 10 minutes
Millet	1½ cups water for 30 minutes	1½–2 cups water for 30 minutes
Whole Oats	2 cups water for 50 minutes	4–5 cups water for 2 hours
Steel-Cut Oats	4 cups water for 30 minutes	4 cups water for 45 minutes

1 cup uncooked grain	Pressure-Cooking	Boiling
Rolled Oats	Do not pressure-cook	3 cups water for 30 minutes
Rice (Brown)	1¼–1½ cups water for 40–50 minutes	1½ cups water for 45–50 minutes

Notes for Basic Grains

- To keep a very low flame for simmering boiled grains and for pressure cooking, a flame deflector may be used.
- The chart on page 50 is a very basic list for cooking grains. You may find that the grain comes out too wet or too dry using these proportions. The ratio of liquid to grain should then be adjusted to suit your personal taste.
- One cup of uncooked grain yields approximately 2–2½ cups of cooked grain.
- Whole-rye berries and whole-wheat berries are usually not cooked alone. A few tablespoons may be added to a pot of rice, in which case they would cook as long as the rice. Because whole wheat and whole rye are so chewy, it is a good idea to soak them in water overnight before cooking.

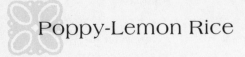

Poppy-Lemon Rice

YIELD: 4 SERVINGS

> 2 cups uncooked brown rice
> 2½ cups water
> ¼–½ teaspoon salt
> *2 tablespoons lemon juice
> 2 tablespoons chopped parsley
> 2 tablespoons finely diced celery
> 3 tablespoons toasted poppy seeds (See page 30 for seed-toasting
> directions.)

Pressure-cook rice, water, and salt for 45 minutes. Use a flame deflector under the pot to reduce the chance of burning your rice. (If boiling is preferred, see Basic Grain Cooking Chart on page 50 for directions.) When completely cooked, stir rest of ingredients into hot rice, and serve.

Tangy Rice Salad

YIELD: 4 SERVINGS

> 1 cup uncooked rice
> 1½ cups water
> ⅛ teaspoon salt
> 1 medium carrot, peeled and diced
> 4 red radishes, quartered
> 4 scallions, sliced

---

*Not recommended on a strict macrobiotic diet.

1 celery stalk, diced

1 tablespoon chopped parsley

*1 tablespoon lemon juice

1 tablespoon white miso

1 tablespoon natto miso

Pressure-cook rice, water, and salt for 45 minutes. (If boiling is preferred, please refer to the Basic Grain Cooking Chart on page 50 for directions.) While rice is cooking, steam carrots and radishes together for about 8 minutes. Combined steamed vegetables, uncooked vegetables, lemon juice, white miso, and natto miso in a medium-sized mixing bowl. Stir vegetable mixture into hot cooked rice, making sure both misos are well blended into rice mixture.

Lightly oil a 3- or 3½-cup mold. Spoon rice salad into mold and press down firmly. Chill for at least 2 hours. Invert onto a plate or an attractive platter to serve.

Shiitake Rice Pilaf

YIELD: 4 SERVINGS

2 cups uncooked brown rice

2½ cups water

¼ teaspoon salt

6 shiitake mushrooms

1 large onion, diced

2 celery stalks, diced

1 teaspoon dark sesame oil

½ cup chopped parsley

1 teaspoon tamari

¼ cup toasted sunflower or pumpkin seeds (See page 30 for seed-toasting directions.)

---

*Not recommended on a strict macrobiotic diet.

Pressure-cook rice, water, salt, and shiitake mushrooms for 45 minutes. (To boil, please refer to Basic Grain Cooking Chart on page 50 for directions.) Sauté onion and celery in oil for about 5 minutes. Add parsley and tamari and sauté for 1 more minute. Stir sautéed vegetables into cooked rice and add seeds. Remove shiitake mushrooms and slice into strips. Remove stems and stir mushroom strips back into rice mixture. The stems may be discarded, as they are difficult to chew. Serve the pilaf hot.

Cleaning Your Grain

Before cooking, grains should be thoroughly cleaned of any dust, sticks or little stones. One way of doing this is to put the grain in a pot, cover it with tap water, and swirl the water and grain together with your hand. Discard the cloudy water into the sink. Do this about three times, removing any debris that may have come out of hiding when you swirled the water. If the grain is particularly dirty, rinse it several times until it is clean. After cleaning the grain, you may prepare it in a number of ways. It can be pressure-cooked, baked, sprouted, boiled, or roasted and then boiled. It can be seasoned with salt only, or with numerous other seasonings. Grains may be cooked with vegetables, condiments, sea vegetables, beans, seeds, or other grains.

Arame Rice Triangles

YIELD: ABOUT 32 TRIANGLES

Basic Triangles
1 cup uncooked arame
2 cups uncooked short grain brown rice
⅛ teaspoon sea salt
3 cups water
2 umeboshi plums or 2 teaspoons umeboshi plum paste

1 medium onion, chopped
2 tablespoons light sesame oil

Dipping Sauce
¼ cup tamari
¼ cup water
1 clove garlic, minced
½ teaspoon grated ginger

Place arame in a strainer, rinse under tap water, and turn over onto a cutting board. Chop arame into ½- to 1-inch pieces and place in a pressure cooker with rice, sea salt, water, and umeboshi plums or plum paste. Pressure-cook for 40 minutes. (If boiling is preferred, follow the same procedure until pressure-cooking instructions. Then, bring rice mixture to boil, lower heat, and simmer for 50 minutes.) In either case, stir chopped onion into hot, cooked rice mixture. (This allows onion to cook just enough to lose its pungency.)

Remove umeboshi plum pits (if using whole plums) and stir umeboshi plum into rice mixture to evenly distribute flavor. Allow mixture to rest in pot for about 10 minutes until it cools slightly. Then, spoon it onto any smooth surface that is at least 9 × 13 inches. A cutting board or baking sheet may be used.

Press and smooth the mixture into the shape of a large rectangle about ¼-inch thick. Make evenly spaced horizontal slices in the arame mixture, as seen in Figure 3.1. Slice diagonally, cutting into triangles with about a 2-inch base, as seen in Figure 3.2.

With a spatula, separate triangles and place them onto an oiled baking sheet. Brush top of each triangle with oil, and broil close to flame for 3–5 minutes. Turn each one over with a spatula, and broil for another 3–5 minutes. Triangles should be slightly crispy and browned.

Combine dipping sauce ingredients. Serve dip in a small bowl with hot, broiled arame rice triangles.

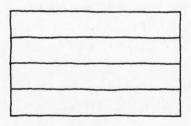

Figure 3.1

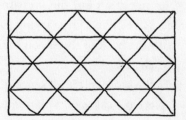

Figure 3.2

Pine Nut Rice Pancakes

YIELD: ABOUT 10 PANCAKES

Pancakes
½ cup short-grain brown rice
½ cup sweet rice
2 cups water
Pinch salt
1 tablespoon flour—rice, corn, or white
8 baby carrots, steamed and diced
1 scallion sliced
2 tablespoons toasted pine nuts
1 tablespoon olive oil

Sauce
¼ cup tamari
3 tablespoons water
2 tablespoons fruit-juice-sweetened apricot preserves

Garnish
Grated ginger

Place rice and water in a pressure cooker. Add salt. Pressure-cook for 35 minutes. Turn off heat and let rice rest until the pressure comes down. Add flour, carrots, scallion, and pine nuts. Heat olive oil in a large frying pan. Place tablespoons of rice mixture into the hot oil. Flatten with the back of the spoon to form each one into a small pancake. Pan-fry for 5 minutes on each side.

To prepare the sauce, place all sauce ingredients in a blender and blend until smooth.

To serve, place pancakes on a platter, with a small spoonful of sauce on top of each one. Sprinkle with grated ginger. Serve remaining sauce on the side, if desired.

Mushroom Grain Squares

YIELD: 4 SERVINGS

> *1 cup uncooked barley*
> *1 cup uncooked brown rice*
> *3½ cups water*
> *⅛ teaspoon sea salt*
> *8 shiitake mushrooms*
> *½ cup chopped scallions*
> *½ cup diced celery*
> *1 teaspoon sesame oil*
> *1 teaspoon prepared mustard*
> *1 tablespoon tamari*
> *2 tablespoons mirin*
> *2 tablespoons umeboshi vinegar*

Pressure-cook barley, brown rice, water, sea salt, and whole shiitake mushrooms for 45 minutes. (To boil, please refer to Basic Grain Cooking Chart on page 50 for directions.) While this is cooking, sauté scallions and celery in oil for about 3 minutes or until vegetables are lightly cooked. Stir sautéed vegetables and mustard into cooked grain. Remove shiitake mushrooms and chop into small pieces, discarding stems. Return to mixture.

Press grain-and-vegetable mixture into a lightly oiled 8-inch square or round baking dish. Combine tamari, mirin, and umeboshi vinegar in a small bowl. Pour this mixture carefully over the top of pressed grain mixture. Bake at 350°F for about 20 minutes.

For a crusty top, place under broiler for about 5 minutes. Cut into squares and serve warm or cool.

Debbie Harrison

Wild Oats Community Market
Andover, Massachusetts

Debbie Harrison is the manager of the bakery department at Wild Oats in Andover, Massachusetts. Her experience, covering a twenty-year span in the field of natural foods and macrobiotic cookery, includes cooking for cancer patients; creating original recipes for the deli case at a downtown Andover health food store; and teaching numerous cooking classes. Her experience also includes cooking for private clients, especially in the field of vegan cookery. Debbie, a trained artist and potter, is also experienced in the art of raising her teen-age daughter.

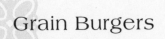

Grain Burgers

by Debbie Harrison
Wild Oats Community Market

YIELDS: 8 BURGERS

6–8 cups cooked short-grain brown rice
1 pound firm tofu
1 large carrot, peeled and grated
1–2 cups cooked chickpeas
½ bunch scallions, sliced
¾ cup toasted sunflower seeds
1 tablespoon dijon mustard
2 tablespoons tamari soy sauce
2 teaspoons herb salt
2 cups cornmeal
Vegetable oil for frying

Mix all above ingredients together, except the cornmeal and oil. Form into patties about palm size. Roll each grain burger in cornmeal. Pan fry in ¼ inch vegetable oil at medium heat until golden brown on both sides. This will require that you turn the burgers after they are brown on the first side. Total cooking time is about 10 minutes. Place hot grain burger on a clean brown paper bag that has been opened to lie flat to absorb any excess oil from frying. Serve warm with dijon mustard or condiment of your choice.

Rice Pilaf

by Julia Ferre
George Ohsawa Macrobiotic Foundation

YIELD: ABOUT 8 CUPS

3 cups uncooked brown rice
1 teaspoon corn oil
1 medium onion, minced
2 medium celery stalks, cut into thin half-rounds
1 medium carrot, peeled and cut into thin quarter-rounds
1 to 2 teaspoons soy sauce
¼ teaspoon sea salt
6 cups boiling water

Preheat oven to 350°F. Wash and drain rice. Place in a dry skillet (no oil) and dry-roast over medium heat. Stir constantly. In about 5 minutes, all the rice will be browned, popped,* and fragrant.

Heat oil in heavy pan over medium heat. Add minced onions and sauté until transparent, 1 to 2 minutes. Add celery and sauté 1 minute. Add carrot and sauté 30 seconds. Remove from heat and add soy sauce.

Place roasted grain, sautéed vegetables, sea salt, and boiling water in a large casserole dish. Cover. Bake for 1 hour.

---

*Rice will make a popping sound while being roasted.

Rice Kayu Bread

by The Kushi Institute

YIELD: 1 LOAF

2 cups whole-wheat flour
⅛–¼ teaspoon sea salt
2 cups soft rice
Sesame oil

Mix flour and sea salt together. Add soft rice and make a ball of dough. (Soft rice is rice that has been cooked with more water than usual—sometimes double the amount. If rice is soft enough, you do not need to add water to make dough. If you use plain, pressure-cooked rice, add a little water to form the ball of dough. Knead dough about 350–400 times. As you are kneading, occasionally sprinkle a little flour on dough to prevent it from sticking to the bowl.

Oil a standard medium-sized loaf pan with a little sesame oil and sprinkle with a little flour—this will prevent bread from sticking to pan. Form dough into loaf shape and place in floured pan. Lightly press edges of dough down to form a rounded-loaf effect.

With a knife, make a shallow slit in top center of dough. Cover loaf with a clean, damp towel.

Place loaf in a warm place, such as the oven with the pilot light or inside lightbulb on, or near a warm radiator. Let dough sit for 8–10 hours, occasionally moistening towel with warm water as it dries out. After the rising period, place dough in oven with temperature set at 200–250°F for about 30 minutes. Increase the temperature to 350°F and continue to bake for about 60–75 minutes longer.

When bread is done, remove from bread pan and place on rack to cool. Slice and serve.

For variation, ¼–½ cup raisins and/or roasted seeds may be kneaded into the dough before it is baked.

The Kushi Institute

Becket, Massachusetts
www.kushiinstitute.org

The Kushi Institute, located in the Berkshire Mountains in Becket, Massachusetts, has been a place of refuge, transformation, and instruction for the many who have been touched by its mission. Established in 1978 by Michio and Aveline Kushi, the Kushi Institute reaches out to the world with its macrobiotic philosophy and practical principles for living.

Michio and Aveline's teachings were inspired by George Ohsawa, a philosopher and writer whose works blended thoughts of traditional Asian medicine with Western traditions. The macrobiotic approach as taught by the Kushi Institute underscores the importance of choosing a diet and lifestyle that are most conducive to physical, emotional, and spiritual wholeness.

Drawing students from many nations, the Kushi Institute is the leading macrobiotic center in the world. Weeklong "Way to Health" programs are offered to individuals seeking a deeper knowledge of macrobiotics for personal-health reasons or to assist in the restoration of the health of another. The "Macrobiotic Career Training Program" instructs students who are interested in pursuing careers in macrobiotic cooking or counseling. The Kushi Institute, with its devoted staff and respected leaders, has touched the world in its mission to motivate and educate with the intent of achieving personal well-being and freedom in order to then touch, teach, and inspire others.

Millet Flat Bread

YIELD: 9 PIECES, 2 INCHES SQUARE

1 cup uncooked millet
2½ cups water

¼ teaspoon sea salt
1 small onion, diced
2 tablespoons toasted poppy or caraway seeds (See page 30 for seed-
toasting directions.)

Bring millet, water, and sea salt to boil in medium-sized saucepan. Lower heat, cover, and simmer for 30 minutes.

Stir diced onion and seeds into warm millet. Cover and let it sit for 5 minutes. (This allows the onion to retain its texture, but to lose its pungency.)

Press warm millet mixture ¼-inch thick onto a 9- × 13-inch baking sheet and let cool. Cut flatbread into sandwich-sized slices. Use for sandwiches, appetizers, or snacks.

Tortillas

by Celeste Skardis

YIELD: 1½ POUNDS OR 4–6 SERVINGS

There are many ways to cook with dried corn—corn muffins, corn bread, cornmeal, hominy grits, tortillas, tostadas, and tacos. The cellulose outer covering must be removed from the corn in order for it to be completely edible. This process is done by cooking the dried corn with water and wood ash. Wood ash can be made from hardwood burned in a clean fireplace or woodstove, from a fire that has been started without newspaper.

The best tortillas are made from white flint corn; the next best from blue corn or dent corn.

Basic Corn
3½ cups dried corn
2 cups water
½ cup finely sifted wood ash (For softer corn, add more wood ash.)

Pressure-cook ingredients for 20 minutes. Let cool in pot so that pressure comes down. Rub skins off kernels and rinse well, discarding skins. If skins don't come off by simply rubbing, add more wood ash and cook for 10 to 15 more minutes in pressure cooker. Cool, and rinse well.

After rinsing the corn, put it in a pressure cooker and add a little less than 2 cups of water. Pressure-cook for 45–55 minutes. Corn should be very soft when done.

Tortillas

Grind cooked corn in a Corona mill or any food mill used for grinding grains, beans, and other foods. With your hands, make balls the size of golf balls with corn until all corn mush is used up. Roll each one out in a flat, circular shape, or press in a tortilla press. Place each one on a hot, oiled, cast-iron pan and cook for only a few seconds. Transfer to a plate or tray and repeat process until all flat corn circles have been cooked.

Tortillas may be served warmed, topped with beans and chopped vegetables; deep-fried, topped with beans and chopped vegetables; or plain, warmed or deep-fried. They also may be cut into pie-shaped wedges, deep-fried, and used as corn chips for snacks, dips, or in any way corn chips are used.

Sprouted Rye Bread

YIELD: 1 SMALL LOAF

> *Large glass jar*
> *Piece of cheesecloth large enough to cover mouth of jar*
> *Rubber band*
> *¾ pound rye berries*
> *1 teaspoon salt*

Place rye berries in large jar. Cover with water and let soak overnight. In the morning, place a double-layered piece of cheesecloth over mouth of jar, and secure it to edge of jar with a rubber band, making a strainer top. Drain water through cheesecloth.

Let rye berries sit overnight at room temperature, turning jar upside down inside a bowl, allowing excess water to drain out. Rinse the berries again in the morning, and let them sit upside down once more overnight. By morning, each rye berry should have a tiny sprout.

Grind sprouts and salt together in food grinder or electric food processor. Grind until berries are the consistency of dough. Knead for 5 minutes into a small 1-inch-high loaf, about 6 inches long and 3 inches wide. Place on any-size oiled baking pan in which the loaf will fit, as it won't expand during cooking. Bake at 300°F for about 2 hours, and cool. The outside will be crusty, while the inside will be very moist and sweet tasting. Refrigerate to store.

Variations

- Use wheat berries instead of rye, or combine the two.
- Knead ½ cup nuts or seeds into dough before baking.
- Knead ½ cup raisins into dough before baking.

Chapati

by Cornellia Aihara
George Ohsawa Macrobiotic Foundation

YIELD: ABOUT 17 CHAPATI, EACH 4 INCHES IN DIAMETER

7 cups finely ground whole-wheat flour
2½ cups warm water (body temperature)
2 teaspoons sea salt

To make dough: Mix sea salt and water in small bowl. Place flour in large bowl. Make a shallow hole in center of flour. Pour salted water into hole all at once. Hold the bowl and with one hand, and, with just the fingers of the other hand, stir in circles—small to large—until all the water is absorbed. Make dough into a ball.

To knead: Knead dough with the heels of the hands. Poke holes in dough with thumbs as you hold dough in both hands. Fold dough over holes and press with heels of hands. Turn flattened dough ¼ turn and repeat kneading process until dough is a little softer than earlobe consistency, and a little more moist than bread dough. It takes about 10 minutes for the gluten to come and the texture to become rubbery.

To rise: Let dough sit 24 hours at room temperature in a bowl covered with a wet towel, or in a porcelain pot covered with a lid.

To form balls: Knead dough a few times in the bowl. Lightly flour your working space. Pinch off small portions of dough and roll them into balls about 2 inches in diameter. Make as many balls as you need for the meal to be served. Roll balls in flour so they are lightly coated.

To roll out: Press down one ball with the heel of the hand until it is ⅓-inch thick, then roll out with a rolling pin or surikogi to 4 or 5 inches in diameter. Roll out only one chapati at a time, and cook immediately.

To cook—Step 1: Heat cast-iron frying pan, griddle, or other heavy skillet until hot. No oil should be used. Place rolled-out chapati in hot frying pan (medium flame) for 1–2 minutes. Small bumps will appear on surface of dough. Push them down lightly with backs of fingers. Turn chapati over and cook 1 minute. Dough will change color from raw gray to cooked tan, but should not start to expand.

Cornellia Aihara

George Ohsawa Macrobiotic Foundation
Vega Study Center
Oroville, California

Cornellia Aihara was born in Japan. It was there that she first studied macrobiotics at George Ohsawa's school. She later moved to the United States and married Herman Aihara, a teacher of macrobiotics. Since 1961, Cornellia has traveled to many parts of the world teaching macrobiotic cooking and philosophy. She has also written several books. Her works include: *The Do of Cooking; Macrobiotic Kitchen; The Calendar Cookbook;* and *Macrobiotic Childcare.*

Cornellia has contributed a recipe for chapati, a round, flat bread that is commonly eaten in India. Of this recipe, she says, "I am especially happy to introduce this chapati recipe because it is an easy-to-make food (with a little practice). Its preparation can be incorporated into a busy daily schedule."

To cook—Step 2: Set gas flame on medium-low. Place chapati on cake rack. Using an oven mitt to protect your hands, hold rack at a 30-degree angle to flame. Make circular motions, allowing flame to heat edges of chapati first. Rotate chapati periodically so every part of its edge has a chance to be nearest the flame. The dough will expand, balloonlike. Continue to cook with circular motions. You will see steam escaping along the edge. Turn over and continue cooking until golden brown. (Note: Sometimes the dough doesn't completely expand. The pocket, formed from the dough expansion, will have formed anyway if all the steam has escaped.)

To keep hot until served: Line a ceramic bowl with a large, wet, terry-cloth towel. Put cooked chapati in bowl and cover with ends of towel. When all chapati are cooked and placed in bowl, cover again with ends of towel. Then, put a lid of aluminum foil over top of bowl and place bowl in warm oven. This method is especially helpful if you are making a lot of chapati.

To store dough: Dough can be refrigerated 5–6 days. Cover to keep it from drying out. It will become slightly softer each day as more gluten comes out. Don't add any flour. This softer dough is actually easier to work with. After 5 days, the dough will smell slightly sour, but when baked, is more sweet and digestible than the chapati made the first 2–3 days.

Recommendations for daily use: Decide how many chapati you want to serve in a week. Make enough dough on a Saturday or Sunday for the week, and keep it in the refrigerator. Make balls, roll out dough, and cook chapati just before each meal or snack. It takes about 5 minutes to make each chapati.

For small children and elderly people: One-third to one-half of the flour used could be replaced with unbleached white flour for a softer, more digestible bread.

Sweet Rice Corn Bread

YIELD: 4 SERVINGS

¾ cup sweet rice
2 cups water
pinch sea salt
1 tablespoon corn oil

½ cup raisins or currants
¼ cup toasted sunflower seeds (See page 30 for seed-toasting directions.)
1 cup cornmeal

Pressure-cook sweet rice, water, and sea salt for 40 minutes. (If boiling is preferred, please refer to Basic Grain Cooking Chart on page 50 for directions.) Combine rest of ingredients with cooked sweet rice and press into an oiled loaf pan. Bake at 400°F, covered with foil, for 30 minutes. Uncover and bake another 15 minutes to slightly brown the top. Slice and serve warm or at room temperature.

Rolled Oat Flat Bread

YIELD: 9 PIECES, 2 INCHES SQUARE

2 cups uncooked rolled oats
¼ teaspoon sea salt
Water to cover—about 3 cups
1 medium onion, chopped
⅓ cup toasted sunflower or sesame seeds (See page 30 for seed-toasting directions.)

In a medium-sized mixing bowl, cover the oats and sea salt with water and set aside for about 30 minutes, or until all the water is absorbed. Add onion and seeds. Spread this thick oat mixture onto an oiled 9- × 13-inch baking sheet so that uncooked flat bread is about ¼–½-inch thick. Bake at 350°F for 45–60 minutes. Serve warm or cool, with a spread or plain.

Variation

- Omit onion and add ⅓ cup raisins instead.

4.

❖ ❖ ❖

Tofu and Tempeh

The world of soy products has expanded tremendously over the past ten years. Tofu and tempeh, and prepared foods derived from these two foods, have introduced the public to a versatile, low-fat, cholesterol-free protein source—the soybean.

Though tofu and tempeh are both created from soybeans, they are very different products. Tofu is a bland, white soybean curd that is usually pressed into one-pound cakes. Tofu's characteristic blandness is actually a plus, as it will absorb the flavor of any marinade, sauce, or seasoning. Its versatility is expanded by its consistency, which may be firm, soft, or silken (silky smooth).

Tempeh, unlike tofu, has a very distinct flavor and consistency. It has a unique flavor and a firm, meatlike consistency. Both tofu and tempeh may be prepared as dips, appetizers, salads, main dishes, and side dishes.

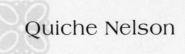

Quiche Nelson

by Nissan Balaban

YIELD: 6–8 SERVINGS

Crust
1 cup whole-wheat flour (rough ground)
1 cup whole-wheat pastry flour (fine ground)
1 cup fine-ground cornmeal
½ teaspoon sea salt
1 teaspoon brewer's yeast
½ cup corn oil
1 cup warm water

Filling
1½ pounds tofu
3 tablespoons raw tahini
2 tablespoons shoyu
1 teaspoon sea salt
½ cup water
2 medium-sized onions
10–15 parsley leaves

In a large bowl, combine whole-wheat flour, pastry flour, cornmeal, sea salt, and brewer's yeast. Pour in oil and, with a fork, mix well. Pour in the water and knead dough for about 5 minutes. Leave to rest, covered, for 30 minutes.

Roll out dough between two sheets of wax paper and place in a 12-inch round pan, pressing up 1-inch borders all around. Pierce the bottom of the crust a few times with a fork. Bake in a preheated oven (400°F) for 15 minutes. Leave to cool.

In a suribachi or blender, mix tofu, tahini, shoyu, sea salt, and water until creamy. Grate onions, chop parsley leaves, and add to mixture, combining well. Pour filling into crust, smoothing top with a spatula. Bake for 45 minutes. To test if done, insert a toothpick into the center. When toothpick comes out dry, quiche is ready.

Dill Cauliflower Sauce over Noodles

YIELD: 4 SERVINGS

1 pound tofu
1 medium onion, chopped
1 teaspoon dried dill or 2 teaspoons fresh dill
1 tablespoon rice vinegar
½ teaspoon sea salt
¼ cup water
2 teaspoons kuzu
1 cup water
1 small head cauliflower, broken into small flowerets—about 3 cups
1 pound flat artichoke or whole-wheat noodles
1 tablespoon toasted poppy seeds (See page 30 for seed-toasting directions.)

Cut tofu into small cubes (about ¼ inch) and drop into boiling water to cover. Boil 2–3 minutes to make tofu easier to digest. Drain cubes and set aside.

Simmer onion, dill, rice vinegar, and sea salt in ¼ cup water until onions are transparent. Dissolve kuzu in 1 cup water and add to pot of vegetables. Stir over medium heat until thickened—about 5 minutes.

Steam cauliflower for about 10 minutes or until lightly cooked. Add cauliflower and tofu to vegetable sauce and keep hot over very low flame. Boil noodles in salted water for about 10 minutes or until tender. Drain and rinse. Toss cooked, warm noodles with poppy seeds. Serve cauliflower sauce over noodles, and garnish with chopped parsley or scallions, if desired.

Marinated Baked Tofu

Yield: 15–20 slices

> *1 pound tofu*
> *¼ cup tamari*
> *¼ cup water*
> *1 teaspoon grated ginger*
> *½ medium onion, diced or grated*
> **1 tablespoon lemon juice*

Slice tofu into pieces approximately ¼ inch thick. Pour rest of ingredients over tofu slices and marinate in a covered container in the refrigerator for several hours or overnight. This process allows the tofu to absorb much of the flavor of the marinade. Place slices on a 9- × 13-inch baking pan, pouring remaining marinade over them. Bake at 350°F for about 20 minutes. The longer it bakes, the drier the tofu will become. Serve warm or cool, with noodles, whole grains, or on sandwiches.

Ginger-Garlic Tofu

Yield: 4 servings

> *1 pound tofu, cut into ½-inch cubes*
> *½ cup water*
> *1 tablespoon tamari*
> *1 teaspoon grated ginger*

---

*Not recommended on a strict macrobiotic diet.

2 tablespoons diced onion
2 cloves garlic, minced

Combine all ingredients in a 2-quart or larger saucepan. Bring to boil, lower heat, and simmer for 15–20 minutes. This allows tofu to absorb all the seasonings. Add a little water if liquid mixture dries out too quickly. Serve warm or cool by itself; mixed with vegetables, grains, or salads; or in sandwiches, soups, or casseroles.

Cabbage with Tofu

Yield: 4 servings

1 small head cabbage, thinly sliced
3 shiitake mushrooms
1 medium onion, thinly sliced
1 pound tofu, cut into ¼-inch cubes
½ cup water
1 tablespoon tamari
1 teaspoon umeboshi vinegar
1 teaspoon mirin

Bring cabbage, shiitake mushrooms, and onion to boil in ½ inch of water. Lower heat, and simmer in a medium-sized covered saucepan for about 10 minutes until vegetables are soft. While vegetables are simmering, drop tofu cubes into a saucepan of ½ cup boiling water, and boil for 1–2 minutes. Drain tofu cubes and purée them in a food mill, or mash them with a fork or potato masher.

Remove shiitake mushrooms, slice and discard tough stems. In a large mixing bowl, combine cooked vegetables, mashed tofu, tamari, umeboshi vinegar, and mirin. Return soft mushrooms to tofu-vegetable mixture. Serve over noodles or a whole grain garnished with chopped scallions, parsley, toasted sesame seeds, or toasted almonds.

Crusty Millet Pizza with Carrot Sauce

YIELD: 4 SERVINGS

This dish involves 3 preparations—the tofu, the crust, and the sauce.

Tofu
1 cup sweet rice, soaked overnight in 2 cups water
Pinch sea salt
½ pound tofu
1 medium onion, finely chopped
2 small umeboshi plums with pits removed, or 1 heaping teaspoon of
    umeboshi plum paste

Pressure-cook rice, soaking water, pinch sea salt, and whole piece of tofu for 20 minutes. Stir hot rice-tofu mixture, onion, and umeboshi in suribachi with a surikogi (pestle) until most of the grains are mashed and consistency becomes sticky. Add ¼–½ cup water and stir a few more minutes to achieve a thinner, more melted-cheese–like consistency. Refrigerate.

Crust
1 cup uncooked millet
2½ cups water
⅛ teaspoon sea salt
1 teaspoon olive oil

Bring millet, water, and sea salt to boil in medium-sized saucepan. Lower heat, cover, and simmer for 30 minutes. Press warm grain onto a round 12-inch pizza pan. A 9- × 12-inch rectangular baking sheet can also be used. Brush millet crust with olive oil and put under broiler for 3–5 minutes, or until light golden brown. Remove from broiler and set aside.

Sauce

4 large carrots or 6 medium carrots, peeled and sliced
1 large onion, chopped
1 teaspoon umeboshi plum paste
2 cloves garlic, minced
¼ teaspoon basil
¼ teaspoon ground bay leaf
¼–½ cup water
1 teaspoon miso

Bring sauce ingredients (except for miso) to boil. Lower heat, cover, and simmer for about 20 minutes until carrots are very soft. Purée all ingredients, including miso, in a food mill. The sauce should have the consistency of thick mayonnaise.

To assemble pizza, spread sauce on top of crust and spread tofu mixture on top of sauce. Add any toppings of your choice, such as raw scallions, sautéed or raw onions, olives, cooked tempeh, seitan, or steamed squash. Bake for 15 minutes at 400°F, or put under broiler for about 5 minutes to brown the top. Serve warm.

Variations

* Add more garlic, thyme, oregano, or marjoram to the sauce.
* Substitute Lasagna sauce on page 81 or Muffin Pizza sauce on page 84 for the carrot sauce.

Ginger Tofu Pie

YIELD: 4 SERVINGS

1 cup uncooked brown rice
1½ cups water with pinch sea salt
4 medium carrots, peeled and grated
2 medium turnips, peeled and grated
1 medium onion, chopped

¼ teaspoon sea salt

1 cup water

½ pound tofu

1 small onion, diced

1 teaspoon grated ginger

1 tablespoon tamari

1 teaspoon light or dark sesame oil

1 tablespoon toasted sesame seeds (See page 30 for seed-toasting directions.)

Pressure-cook rice, water, and sea salt for 45 minutes. (To boil, please refer to Basic Grain Cooking Chart on page 50 for directions.) While rice is cooking, bring carrots, turnips, medium onion, and ¼ teaspoon sea salt to boil in ½ cup water. Lower heat, and simmer for 10 minutes until vegetables are soft. Set aside.

Boil tofu, small onion, ginger, tamari, and ½ cup water over medium heat for about 5 minutes. Then, purée in a food mill placed over a large bowl. Put 1 cup of rice through the food mill placed over the same bowl. Some of the grains will go through and some will just get mashed.

Combine tofu, ingredients tofu was cooked with, and whole and partially puréed rice. Moisten your hands with water and form a crust using your hands to mold the mixture onto a 9-inch pie plate. Brush crust with oil and put under broiler for 5 minutes. Remove from broiler and fill crust with carrot, turnip, and onion mixture. Sprinkle sesame seeds over filling and bake at 350°F for 15 minutes. Serve hot.

Hambulghur Helper

by Jessica Porter

YIELD: 8 SERVINGS

¼ cup toasted sesame oil

8 ounces of tempeh, sliced into bite-sized cubes

2 tablespoons toasted sesame oil

1 medium onion, diced
⅛ teaspoon sea salt
1 large carrot, cut into matchsticks
2 cups bulghur wheat
1 cup whole-wheat rotini or elbow noodles
5 cups water
3 tablespoons shoyu
2 tablespoons mirin
⅛ teaspoon brown rice vinegar
1 cob of corn
2 stalks of celery, diced

In a large frying pan, heat ¼ cup sesame oil over medium heat. When oil is hot (but not smoking) add tempeh, frying the cubes until browned and crispy. Remove from heat and let drain on paper towel. Set aside.

In a 6-quart pot, heat 2 tablespoons of sesame oil over medium heat. Add onions and salt and sauté until translucent. Add carrots and sauté for a few minutes. Pour in bulghur wheat and noodles, stirring them into vegetables. Fold in tempeh.

Mix water, shoyu, mirin, and vinegar all together in a bowl and pour into bulghur wheat mixture. Bring to a boil uncovered. Reduce flame to low and cover. Let simmer 15 minutes. Remove the kernels from the ear of corn. Add corn and celery to the pot. Cook for 5 more minutes. Remove from heat and let sit a couple of minutes to prevent sticking. Serve with steamed or boiled greens.

Tofu Shish Kebab

YIELD: 4 SERVINGS

¼ cup tamari
1½ teaspoons grated ginger
1 tablespoon rice vinegar

1 tablespoon rice syrup

1 cup water

1 tablespoon mirin

1 pound tofu, cut into 1-inch cubes

1 tablespoon kuzu

2 cups broccoli flowerets

2 cups carrot peeled and cut into chunks

2 cups turnip peeled and cut into wedges

1 tablespoon toasted sesame seeds (See page 30 for seed-toasting directions.)

Bring tamari, ginger, rice vinegar, rice syrup, water, and mirin to boil in medium-sized saucepan. Add tofu cubes, lower heat, and simmer tofu in this mixture for 15 minutes. Remove tofu with chopsticks or a fork and set aside. Dissolve kuzu in a small amount of cool tamari mixture, and stir it back into that mixture. Stir over medium heat for about 5 minutes, until thickened and clear, and set aside.

Steam broccoli, carrots, and turnips until they are lightly cooked, but still firm, and set aside.

Skewer tofu and vegetables on stainless-steel or bamboo skewers, alternating tofu with vegetables so that each skewer looks attractive and colorful. Spoon tamari-kuzu sauce over each skewer and broil for a few minutes until hot and glazed with sauce. Remove from broiler, sprinkle with toasted sesame seeds, and serve with rice.

Tofu, Pasta, and Olives

Yield: 4 servings

1 pound soft tofu

2 medium onions, diced

2 cups chopped kale

2 tablespoons olive oil

3 tablespoons light miso
½ teaspoon ground bay leaf
1 cup ripe black olives or ¼ cup green olives
1 pound udon, artichoke, whole-wheat, or soba noodles

Drop tofu in medium-sized saucepan of boiling water to cover for 2–3 minutes. Remove from water and set aside. Sauté onions and kale in oil. Put tofu, onion, and kale in a suribachi and grind to a paste consistency. Add miso and bay leaf and grind until blended. Slice olives, stir them in, and set aside.

Boil noodles for about 10 minutes or until tender. Combine tofu mixture with hot pasta and serve.

If desired, pasta-and-tofu mixture may be placed in a 9-inch square or round baking dish and put under broiler for 3–5 minutes before serving. This will form a light, crusty topping.

Tofu Grilled "Cheesy" Sandwiches

YIELD: 2 SANDWICHES

1 small onion, diced
½ teaspoon light sesame oil
¼ tofu, crumbled
1 piece mochi, 2 inches square and ½-inch high, cut into very small
    pieces or grated
2 tablespoons water
1 teaspoon umeboshi plum paste
⅛ teaspoon turmeric
1 teaspoon prepared mustard (such as French's)
4 slices sourdough bread
Oil to brush pan for grilling sandwiches

Sauté onion in oil for a few minutes until pearly white. Add tofu, mochi, and water. Sauté for a few minutes more and add umeboshi plum paste, turmeric, and mustard. Stir continuously for 1–2 minutes until mixture becomes sticky.

Remove mochi mixture from heat and spread evenly on 2 slices of bread, then top each with another slice of bread.

Grill sandwiches on a lightly oiled pan over medium heat for about 5 minutes on each side or until each side is toasted. Slice and serve hot.

Variations

- After spreading bread with mochi mixture, add sliced pickles, top with the other slice of bread, and grill.
- Put mochi mixture in a blender for a creamier texture.
- Add 1 tablespoon tahini to mochi mixture for a richer taste.

Fettuccine Lermano

YIELD: 2–3 SERVINGS

¼ pound tofu

2 cloves garlic, minced

2 tablespoons olive oil

1 umeboshi plum (pit removed) or 1 teaspoon umeboshi plum paste

½ teaspoon sea salt

¾–1 cup water

¼ teaspoon dry mustard

8 ounces artichoke, whole-wheat, or spinach fettuccine

¼ cup chopped parsley

2 tablespoons chopped green olives

Boil tofu in water to cover for 2 minutes, drain, and set aside. Purée tofu, garlic, oil, umeboshi plum, sea salt, water, and mustard in a suribachi, blender, or food processor until smooth. Heat tofu mixture in a medium-sized saucepan over a very low flame. While sauce is heating, boil fettuccine for 8–10 minutes or until tender. Toss fettuccine, tofu sauce, parsley, and olives together in large pot or mixing bowl. Transfer to platter and serve hot.

Lasagna

YIELD: 4–6 SERVINGS

Basic Lasagna
12 ounces whole-wheat, artichoke, or spinach lasagna noodles

Filling
2 pieces mochi, about 2 inches square and ½-inch high
1 pound tofu
½ small onion, chopped
2 umeboshi plums (pits removed), or 2 heaping teaspoons of umeboshi plum paste
¼ teaspoon sea salt
About ½ cup water

Sauce
2–3 cloves garlic, minced
1 tablespoon olive oil
1 large onion, diced
4 large carrots, peeled and sliced
½ small beet, peeled and diced
1 bay leaf
¼ teaspoon oregano, thyme, or basil
5 mushrooms, sliced
5 green olives, sliced
1 teaspoon rice vinegar
1 teaspoon dark miso

In a large pot, boil lasagna for about 15 minutes or until tender, stirring frequently to prevent sticking. Drain and set aside.

Cut mochi into small squares and bake in 400°F oven for about 10 minutes or until soft, but not crispy. Purée baked mochi, tofu, onion, umeboshi, sea salt, and water in food processor or sturdy blender to achieve the consistency of hot, melted cheese, adding more water if necessary. Set filling aside.

To prepare sauce, sauté garlic in olive oil in a 4-quart or larger pressure cooker for a couple of minutes (you can use a separate pan, but why wash an extra pan?) Add onion, carrots, beet, and herbs. Add about ½ cup water, and pressure-cook for 15 minutes. Mash cooked vegetable mixture with a potato masher or purée in a food mill or blender. Return mixture to pot, stir in sliced mushrooms, olives, rice vinegar, and miso, and set aside.

To assemble lasagna, spoon 2–3 tablespoons of sauce on the bottom of a 9- × 13- × 2-inch baking dish, and cover with lasagna strips placed side by side. Spread with a layer of filling, then with a layer of sauce. Repeat process until all lasagna is used up, topping last layer with filling. Bake in 375°F oven for about 30 minutes or until hot. Cut into large squares and serve.

Tofu Casserole

by Spring Street Natural Restaurant

YIELD: 6 SERVINGS

2 pounds tofu
1½ cups raw whole almonds
3 tablespoons tamari
1 cup water
3 cloves garlic
1 quart mushrooms, sliced
2 cups onions, diced into ¾-inch pieces
2 tablespoons oil
⅓ cup tamari

1 teaspoon sea salt
2 tablespoons thyme
2 tablespoons basil
½ teaspoon pepper
1½ quarts chopped, fresh spinach
Sesame seeds

Place tofu in a colander and allow to drain. Spread almonds on a cookie sheet and bake at 375°F for 10–12 minutes until the interior is lightly browned and crunchy. Toss with 3 tablespoons tamari immediately after removing from oven. Allow almonds to cool. When cool, purée with water and garlic in food processor (small almond chunks are okay).

Sauté mushrooms and onions in oil until mushrooms release some of their water (approximately 10 minutes). Add tamari and seasonings, and cook on a very low flame another 10 minutes. Let cool.

Crumble drained tofu (tofu must be well drained to reach desired consistency) and combine with *all* ingredients, except sesame seeds, in large bowl. Spoon into oiled individual casseroles. Sprinkle generously with sesame seeds. Bake in 400°F oven for 12–15 minutes, until hot in the center.

Note: Flavor is greatly enhanced by fresh herbs. Texture should be firm and moist, not crumbly. If individual casseroles are not available, bake in large baking dish at 350°F for 20–30 minutes, or until hot in the center.

Spring Street Natural Restaurant

New York, New York

The Spring Street Natural Restaurant is located on a busy corner along the main route in lower Manhattan, between the East Village and Soho.

The restaurant does not serve red meat, frozen foods, or chemical or artificial ingredients. Everything is made to order, from scratch. The restaurant features fresh fish, poultry, pasta, and vegetarian dishes.

Larry's Favorite—Muffin Pizza

YIELD: 4 SERVINGS

Tofu-Rice Topping
2 cups leftover rice or soft rice (pressed into measuring cup)
¼ pound tofu
1 tablespoon tahini
1 large or 2 small umeboshi plums (pits removed)
½ small onion, chopped
*Water to achieve "cheesy" consistency (will vary depending on
    how moist the rice is)*

Sauce
2 cloves garlic, minced
½ small onion, finely chopped
*½ green pepper, finely chopped
1 teaspoon olive oil
¼ teaspoon basil
Pinch cayenne pepper
*6 ounces tomato paste
½ cup water
¼ teaspoon dark miso

Muffins
4 whole-wheat English muffins, sliced in half

Garnishes
Green or black olives, sliced
Cooked tempeh, tofu, or seitan pieces

---

*Not recommended on a strict macrobiotic diet.

Mushrooms, sliced
Onions, sliced
*Green pepper, sliced

Cook extra rice or soft rice the day before you plan to prepare this recipe. Purée tofu-rice topping ingredients in a blender, food processor, or suribachi, adding enough water to achieve a melted-cheese-like consistency, and set aside.

Sauté garlic, onion, and green pepper in olive oil in a medium-sized saucepan. Add basil, cayenne pepper, tomato paste, and water. Bring to boil, lower heat, and simmer for 10 minutes or until vegetables are very soft. Turn off heat, stir in miso, and set aside.

Place 8 muffin halves on a 9- × 13-inch baking sheet in preheated 400°F oven for 15 minutes. Remove lightly toasted muffins from the oven. Top each one with a heaping tablespoon of sauce, a heaping tablespoon of tofu-rice topping, and any of the garnishes you desire. Return muffin pizzas to 400°F oven and bake for 15 more minutes or until pizza is hot and bubbly.

Tempeh-Vegetable Combo

YIELD: 4 SERVINGS

1 8-ounce package tempeh, cut into 1-inch cubes
1 tablespoon dark sesame oil.
1½ cups water
2 tablespoons tamari
2 teaspoons grated ginger
1 piece kombu, 4 inches long
1 bay leaf
2 medium yellow squash, thickly sliced
3 medium carrots, peeled and sliced
2 medium onions, thickly sliced

---

*Not recommended on a strict macrobiotic diet.

1 tablespoon kuzu, dissolved in ½ cup water
*1 tablespoon rice vinegar
1 tablespoon chopped parsley

Sauté tempeh cubes in oil in a large frying pan until golden brown. Add water, tamari, ginger, kombu, and bay leaf. Bring to boil, lower heat, and simmer uncovered for about 30 minutes. The liquid should bubble a little, but not boil rapidly, and little or no liquid should be left in the pan when done.

Add vegetables and kuzu dissolved in ½ cup water. Simmer for 10–15 more minutes, stirring often, until vegetables are soft and sauce has thickened. Discard bay leaf and stir in rice vinegar. Remove kombu, slice, and return to pot. Garnish with chopped parsley and serve hot with a whole grain or noodles.

Sauerkraut and Tempeh

by Muriel Crisara

YIELD: 4 SERVINGS

1 pound tempeh
1 tablespoon light or dark sesame oil
1 large jar sauerkraut
1 cup spring water
1 teaspoon barley malt
¼ teaspoon caraway seeds
2 tablespoons kuzu, dissolved in ¼ cup water

In large frying pan, brown tempeh in oil on both sides for about ½ hour. Cut tempeh into bite-sized chunks. Place sauerkraut in 2-quart or larger saucepan with spring water, barley malt, and caraway seeds. Add tempeh and simmer for about 1 hour. Add a little more water while cooking if mixture gets too dry. Stir dissolved kuzu into simmering tempeh mixture to thicken. Serve hot, with fresh rye bread.

---

*Not recommended on a strict macrobiotic diet.

5.

Seitan

Seitan is often called "wheat meat" because it is a chewy, meatlike food made from wheat gluten. Wheat gluten is the part of the wheat flour that is left over after eliminating the starch and bran. This is done through a simple process of kneading wheat flour dough and rinsing it several times. The raw wheat gluten may then be boiled or baked with various seasonings in order to create the desired texture and flavor. Sometimes it is fried after being boiled. This creates one more variation in seitan cookery.

The few seitan recipes included here are a small sample of the flavors, consistencies, textures, shapes, and serving styles that are possible to achieve when cooking with seitan. From burgers, roasts, steaks, and loaves to chili, barbequed seitan, seitan noodle soup, and shepherd's pie, seitan can satisfy your desire for the chewiness of meat, as well as your demand for healthful, low-fat, chemical-free cookery.

Seitan Cutlets with Onion-Mushroom Gravy

by Helga Newmark

YIELD: 4 SERVINGS

2 teaspoons light or dark sesame oil
2 cloves garlic, minced
2 large onions, finely sliced
2 cups sliced mushrooms
7 cups water
¼ cup tamari
2 bay leaves
2 cups raw seitan, sliced into 10 cutlets
½ teaspoon sage
½ cup seitan starch water (or 2 tablespoons of either unbleached white
  flour, kuzu root starch, or arrowroot)
1 teaspoon dark miso, puréed in 2 tablespoons water

Heat oil in large skillet or frying pan and sauté garlic, onions, and mushrooms, stirring constantly. Add water, tamari, and bay leaves, and bring to boil. Add raw seitan cutlets and return to boil. Add sage, cover, and simmer over medium-low heat for 40 minutes. Seitan will expand during cooking.

Pour seitan starch water evenly over cutlets, stir gently, cover, and simmer over low heat for 10 minutes to make gravy. If gravy is not thick enough, add more starch water. Add miso purée and simmer for 2–3 more minutes before serving.

Shepherd's Pie

by Jacqueline Wayne

YIELD: 4–6 SERVINGS

1 cup millet
1 medium-sized head cauliflower, cut in large pieces
1½ cups water
Pinch sea salt
12 ounces or 2 cups seitan, cut into cubes
5 ears fresh corn
¼ cup chopped parsley
3–4 tablespoons soy sauce (tamari or shoyu)

Place washed millet and cauliflower pieces in a 4-quart or larger pressure cooker. Add water and salt. Place over high flame and bring to pressure. Turn down flame and pressure-cook for 15 minutes. While millet mixture is cooking, put cubed seitan into the bottom of a casserole dish.

Husk corn and cut off kernels. Layer corn on top of seitan. Remove millet mixture from pot and place in bowl. Mash with fork or potato masher until mixture resembles mashed potatoes. Add chopped parsley and mix. Layer mashed millet mixture over corn. Smooth the top and poke a few small holes on top. Sprinkle on soy sauce. (This makes the top crispy.) Bake at 350°F for 30–40 minutes.

Stir-Fried Seitan and Noodles

YIELD: 4 SERVINGS

*½ recipe raw seitan (To prepare, see recipe for Seitan Wellington on
    page 92–93, but use 5 cups of flour instead of 10.)*
1 piece kombu, 6 inches long
Water to cover seitan
2 tablespoons tamari
1 bay leaf
1½-inch slice ginger
1 pound udon, artichoke, or somen noodles
1–2 tablespoons dark or light sesame oil
1 large or 2 small carrots, peeled and sliced into matchsticks
1–2 tablespoons tamari
5 scallions, cut into long, thin strips
*2 tablespoons toasted sesame, pumpkin, or sunflower seeds (See page 30
    for seed-toasting directions.)*

Flatten ball of raw seitan to about ½-inch high on cutting board and cut into strips. In a 2-quart or larger saucepan, place a piece of kombu, seitan strips, water to cover, 2 tablespoons of tamari, bay leaf, and ginger. Simmer uncovered for 30 minutes. There should be a few bubbles in simmering water mixture, but do not let seitan boil, or the texture will be spongy instead of firm.

While seitan is cooking, boil noodles. The udon and artichoke should take about 10 minutes, while the somen should take about 7–8 minutes. Drain noodles and set aside.

When seitan is cooked, remove it from broth with chopsticks or a slotted spoon, and set aside. Refrigerate the broth, to be used for a soup or stew stock.

In a large wok or frying pan, heat 2 tablespoons oil. Sauté carrots and seitan together for about 10 minutes, or until carrots are soft. Add noodles and continue to sauté, stirring often, until noodles are hot. Add tamari and scallions and stir 1 more minute. Scallions should be bright green and only slightly cooked, but not raw tasting. Serve hot, sprinkled with toasted seeds.

Variation

- If available, purchase cooked seitan. Cut it into strips and stir-fry as the recipe indicates. This will cut down on preparation time.

Glazed Sesame-Seitan Rolls

YIELD: 4 SERVINGS

1 large carrot, quartered lengthwise
1 recipe raw seitan (see Seitan Wellington recipe on pages 92–93)
1 piece kombu, 4 inches long
Water to cover seitan
1 bay leaf
2 shiitake mushrooms
2 tablespoons tamari
1 large broccoli stalk, cut into chunks
5 small boiling onions, peeled
1 tablespoon kuzu, dissolved in ¼ cup water
2 tablespoons toasted sesame seeds, partially ground in a suribachi (See
*   page 30 for seed-toasting directions.)*

Cut carrot sticks into 2-inch pieces and set aside. Divide seitan into 16 to 20 pieces. Flatten each piece into a rectangular shape with your hands, put a carrot in center of each, and roll up seitan to enclose carrot, pressing seitan to the carrot so it doesn't unravel when cooked. Repeat process until all the seitan and carrot pieces are used up.

Put kombu on bottom of a 3-quart or larger saucepan. Add seitan, water to cover, bay leaf, shiitake mushrooms, and tamari. Simmer uncovered for 30 minutes. While seitan is simmering, steam broccoli until it is cooked, but still firm, and set aside.

After seitan is cooked, remove bay leaf and discard. Much of the water will be cooked out, but there should still be about 2 inches left in bottom of pot. If water is completely gone, add enough to equal about 2 inches from the bottom. Stir in onions and kuzu, and continue simmering for 5 more minutes until sauce thickens. Stir in steamed broccoli and sesame seeds. At this point, there will be very little liquid left in the pot, and the seitan and vegetables will be covered with a shiny glaze. Serve hot.

Seitan Wellington

YIELD: 4–6 SERVINGS

Seitan
10 cups whole-wheat flour,
   or 6 cups whole-wheat and
   4 cups unbleached white flour
About 4½ cups water
Water for rinsing
1 piece kombu, 4 inches long
3 tablespoons tamari
2 bay leaves
1 teaspoon onion powder
1 large or 2 small cloves garlic, peeled

Millet Mixture
1 cup uncooked millet
1 medium cauliflower, cut into small pieces
1 large onion, chopped
⅛ teaspoon sea salt
2½ cups water

Glaze

2 teaspoons kuzu

1 cup water, or liquid from cooked seitan

1 tablespoon tamari

1 teaspoon grated ginger

1 tablespoon light or dark sesame oil

To make seitan, put flour into a large bowl, stirring in enough water to make a kneadable dough (usually water is a little less than half the amount of flour). You should now have a ball of dough ready to be kneaded.

Knead dough for about 5 minutes. Put ball of dough in a bowl, cover with water, and let it rest for about 15 minutes. After 15 minutes, begin kneading out the starch and the bran. Knead dough in a bowl of water in the sink until the water turns a milky white—that is the starch coming out. Drain milky water, cover with fresh water, and knead again until soaking water becomes milky white. Repeat process, alternating between warm and cool water each time you use fresh water, until kneading water is almost clear. You will wind up with a ball of glutenous dough that is considerably smaller than the 10 cups of flour you started with. This is raw seitan ready to be cooked.

In this recipe, the entire ball of seitan will be used. Put piece of kombu in bottom of 3-quart or larger saucepan. Add whole piece of seitan, water to cover, 3 tablespoons tamari, 2 bay leaves, 1 teaspoon onion powder, and 1 large or 2 small cloves of garlic. Simmer for 1½ hours. Do not boil. The longer and slower the seitan cooks, the denser the texture will be. When cooked, remove seitan from pot and put on baking sheet to cool.

Bring millet, cauliflower, onion, salt, and 2½ cups of water to boil. Lower heat, cover, and simmer for 30 minutes. Purée this mixture through a food mill. After it cools slightly, use your hands to shape it around the ball of seitan. Try to mold it into a rounded smooth shape, almost like a turkey breast.

In a small saucepan, dissolve kuzu in either 1 cup water or 1 cup of leftover liquid from cooked seitan. Add tamari, ginger, and sesame seed oil. Stir over medium heat until the glaze thickens into a transparent gel. Cover entire roast with glaze, and bake at 350°F for 1 hour. If desired, garnish with carrot flowers and parsley or scallions. Slice and serve hot.

Serve leftovers on sandwiches with mustard and sauerkraut or dill pickles.

6.

❈ ❈ ❈

Vegetables

There is such a variety of vegetables to choose from! What an amazing choice you have when it comes to vegetable selections, combinations, and preparations. Vegetables may be included in breakfast, lunch, dinner, dessert, snacks, and appetizers. They can be boiled, baked, fried, sautéed, steamed, pickled, broiled, or eaten raw.

Vegetables are included in nearly all the recipes in this book, but this chapter focuses on recipes that feature primarily land vegetables, sea vegetables, beans, and combinations of these. It is amazing to think that you can serve delicious vegetables every day and rarely prepare the exact same dish twice.

Tamari-Topped Squash

Yield: 4–6 servings

Basic Stuffed Squash
½ cup uncooked azuki beans
¾ cup uncooked sweet rice
¾ cup short-grain brown rice
⅛ teaspoon sea salt
3½ cups water
3 medium acorn squash, cut in half and seeds removed
1 teaspoon dried dill or 2 teaspoon fresh dill
2 scallions, chopped
2 tablespoons toasted sunflower seeds (See page 30 for seed-toasting
  directions.)
1 tablespoon chopped parsley
1 medium onion, diced

Sauce
2 cups water
1 tablespoon kuzu
2 tablespoons tamari

Pressure-cook beans, rice, sea salt, and water for 50 minutes. If boiling, bring ingredients to boil, lower heat, and simmer for about 1 hour. While grain mixture is cooking, steam squash halves for 15 minutes, place them on a 9- × 13-inch baking sheet, and set aside. Combine cooked grain mixture with dill, scallions, seeds, parsley, and onion. Spoon this grain mixture into squash centers, dividing it evenly among the 6 halves.

Combine sauce ingredients in a small saucepan, thoroughly dissolving the kuzu in the liquid. Stir over medium heat until thickened and clear. Pour a small portion of sauce over each stuffed squash. Bake at 350°F for 20 minutes, until squash is hot and soft, and serve.

Variations

- Instead of using ½ cup uncooked beans, use 1 cup of leftover beans.
- Instead of using 1½ cups of uncooked rice, use 3 cups of cooked rice (measured by pressing the grain into the container).
- Substitute millet for part of the rice.

COOKING BEANS

Most of the recipes in this book that include beans refer to pressure-cooking the beans. However, beans can also be boiled. The following chart can be used as a guide both for boiling and pressure-cooking beans. When beans are boiled, bring water and beans to boil, then simmer for the time suggested on this chart. When soaked beans are mentioned in the pressure-cooking column, this means beans that have been soaked for eight hours or longer.

Basic Bean Cooking Chart

1 cup beans	Pressure-cooking	Boiling
Azuki Beans	*Soaked:* 2½ cups water for 30 minutes *Unsoaked:* 3 cups water for 45 minutes	3 cups water for 45 minutes 3½ cups water for 50–60 minutes
Black Soybeans	*Soaked:* 3 cups water for 1½ hours *Unsoaked:* 4 cups water for 2–3 hours	4 cups water for 4 hours 4 cups water for 6–7 hours
Black Turtle Beans	*Soaked:* 2½–3 cups water for 50 minutes *Unsoaked:* 3 cups water for 60 minutes	3½ cups water for 2–3 hours 4 cups water for 3–4 hours

Basic Bean Cooking Chart *(continued)*

1 cup beans	Pressure-cooking	Boiling
Chickpeas	*Soaked:* 3 cups water for 1½ hours *Unsoaked:* 4 cups water for 2 hours	4 cups water for 2–3 hours 4 cups water for 4–5 hours
Kidney Beans Cannelloni Beans	*Soaked:* 3 cups water for 50 minutes *Unsoaked:* 4 cups water for 1½ hours	3 cups water for 1½–2 hours 4 cups water for 2½–3 hours
Lentils	*Soaked:* 2½ cups water for 20 minutes *Unsoaked:* 3 cups water for 30 minutes	3 cups water for 35 minutes 3 cups water for 45 minutes
Lima Beans	*Soaked:* 3 cups water for 30 minutes *Unsoaked:* 3 cups water for 45 minutes	3 cups water for 1 hour 3½ cups water for 2 hours
Navy Beans	*Soaked:* 3 cups water for 40 minutes *Unsoaked:* 3½ cups water for 50 minutes	3 cups water for 1 hour 4 cups water for 1½–2 hours
Pinto Beans	*Soaked:* 3 cups water for 50 minutes *Unsoaked:* 3½ cups water for 1–1½ hours	3 cups water for 2 hours 4 cups water for 3 hours

1 cup beans	Pressure-cooking	Boiling
Soybeans	*Soaked:* 3 cups water for 1 hour *Unsoaked:* 4 cups water for 2 hours	4 cups water for 3 hours 4 cups water for 5 hours
Split Peas	*Soaked:* not necessary *Unsoaked:* 3 cups water for 30 minutes	3 cups water for 45–50 minutes

Notes for Basic Beans

- One cup of dry, uncooked beans yields about 2½ cups of cooked beans.
- Dry-roasting long-cooking beans, such as black soybeans, can reduce cooking time to 30–40 minutes.
- Soaking refers to an 8-hour or longer time span.
- If pressure-cooking soybeans, black soybeans, or split peas, please note that they have a tendency to foam and clog the vent. Be sure to fill your pressure cooker to no more than 50 percent capacity.
- Many people have found that boiling beans for about 10 minutes before pressure-cooking reduces the total cooking time and increases the digestibility of the beans. I would recommend using this method.
- Adding a piece of kombu also increases the digestibility of beans.

Holiday Green Bean and Squash Casserole

Yield: 6 servings

4 cups butternut or buttercup squash, peeled and cubed
2 cups cut green beans
1 cup + 2 tablespoons sweetened plain soy milk
1 tablespoon kuzu
1 tablespoon tamari
¼ teaspoon onion powder
¼ teaspoon garlic powder
½ cup pecan halves
20 organic corn chips

Steam squash cubes and green beans in a medium-sized saucepan or steamer for about 10–15 minutes or until soft. Place vegetable mixture in a 1½- or 2-quart lightly oiled casserole dish. In a small saucepan, combine the soy milk, kuzu, tamari, onion powder, and garlic powder. Stir until the kuzu is dissolved. Place over medium heat and stir until thickened. Pour soy-milk mixture over the steamed vegetables. Place the pecans and corn chips in a blender and blend to the consistency of bread crumbs. Sprinkle over the casserole. Bake at 350°F for 10–15 minutes or until the topping is lightly browned.

Subtly Sweet Chickpea Stew

Yield: 4 servings

1 cup uncooked chickpeas
3½ cups water
1 piece kombu, 4 inches long

1 bay leaf
3 shiitake mushrooms
1 clove garlic, minced
1 cup chopped onion or 1 large onion, chopped
1 teaspoon dark sesame oil
1 pound broccoli, cut in chunks
1 tablespoon kuzu
¼ cup water
1 tablespoon currants
1 tablespoon tamari or to taste

Pressure-cook chickpeas, water, kombu, bay leaf, and shiitake mushrooms in a 4-quart or larger pressure cooker for 1½ hours, or until soft. (To boil instead of pressure cooking, please refer to Basic Bean Cooking Chart on page 98 for directions, and proceed with the rest of the recipe as it is written.)

Sauté garlic and onion in oil until golden brown and set aside. Lightly steam broccoli until cooked, but still firm, and set aside. Dissolve kuzu in ¼ cup of water and set aside.

When chickpeas are done, remove the bay leaf, kombu, and mushrooms. Slice kombu and mushrooms into small pieces and return them to the pot. Discard bay leaf. Add sautéed garlic and onion, currants, tamari, and kuzu. Stir over medium heat for about 10 minutes, until stew mixture thickens. Add broccoli and cook a few more minutes, or just until broccoli is hot. Serve over grain.

Lemony Lentil Loaf

Yield: 1 loaf or 4 servings

1 cup uncooked lentils
3 cups water
1 piece kombu, 4 inches long
1 cup cooked rice or other grain (pressed into measuring container)
1 tablespoon miso

1 clove garlic, minced
*3 tablespoons lemon juice
1 medium onion, finely chopped
1 teaspoon grated ginger

Pressure-cook lentils, water, and kombu in a 4-quart or larger pressure cooker for 30 minutes. (If boiling instead of pressure cooking, please refer to Basic Bean Cooking Chart on page 98 for directions.) In either case, lentils should be very soft when done.

Remove kombu from pot of cooked lentils, cut it into small pieces, and return to pot. Stir remaining ingredients into cooked lentils, making sure seasonings are evenly distributed. Press lentil mixture into a lightly oiled loaf pan and bake at 350°F for 20–30 minutes. Serve plain, with a sauce, or on sandwiches.

For appropriate sauce recipes, see cooking ingredients and instructions from the following: Crusty Millet Pizza with Carrot Sauce on pages 74–75; Buckwheat Cabbage Rolls on pages 111–12; Saucy Topped Chickpea Patties on pages 104–05; and Enchiladas on pages 105–107.

Creamy Carrots in a Lentil Crust

YIELD: 4 SERVINGS

1 cup uncooked lentils
½ cup uncooked barley
4 cups water
1 piece kombu, 4 inches long
1 bay leaf
8 medium carrots, peeled and sliced
2 medium onions, sliced
pinch sea salt
¼ cup water
1 tablespoon barley miso
3 scallions, sliced

---

*Not recommended on a strict macrobiotic diet.

Pressure-cook lentils, barley, 4 cups water, kombu, and bay leaf for 45 minutes. (If boiling, bring lentils, barley, water, kombu, and bay leaf to boil, lower heat, and simmer for 50 minutes.) While lentil mixture is cooking, steam carrots and onions with pinch of sea salt for 15 minutes, or until soft. Purée in a food mill, adding ¼ cup water, and set aside.

When done, lentil mixture should be thick and somewhat dry. Remove bay leaf from cooked lentils and discard. Remove kombu, cut into small pieces, and return kombu to pot. Thoroughly blend miso into cooked lentil mixture and let it cool. To form pie crust, press cooled lentil mixture onto bottom and sides of an unoiled 9-inch plate. Fill with carrot-onion purée and top with scallions. Serve as is, baked at 350°F for about 30 minutes, or put under broiler for 5 minutes to form a crusty topping.

Sweet Navy Beans

YIELD: 4 SERVINGS

1 cup uncooked navy beans
3 cups water
1 piece kombu, 4 inches long
2 medium carrots, peeled and thinly sliced
1 large onion, diced
1 teaspoon grated ginger
3–4 tablespoons barley malt
1 tablespoon tamari

Pressure-cook navy beans, water, and kombu for 50–60 minutes. (To boil instead of pressure-cooking, please refer to Basic Bean Cooking Chart on page 98 for directions.) While beans are cooking, steam carrots and onion until they are very soft—about 20 minutes—purée them in a food mill, and set aside.

When beans are done, drain broth and save it for soup stock. Remove kombu, dice, and return it to beans. Stir ginger, barley malt, tamari, and carrot purée into beans. You will now have a thick, saucy bean mixture. Simmer over low flame for 5 more minutes to permit flavors to thoroughly blend together. Serve hot or cool, with grains.

Saucy Topped Chickpea Patties

YIELD: 4 SERVINGS

Patties
1 cup uncooked chickpeas
4 cups water
1 piece kombu, 4 inches long
2 bay leaves
½ cup uncooked millet
1 cup water
¼ teaspoon sea salt
1 carrot, peeled and grated
1 onion, chopped
1 scallion, chopped
1 tablespoon tamari

Sauce
2 tablespoons mellow barley miso
*2 tablespoons lemon juice or rice vinegar
1 scallion, chopped
2 tablespoons water

Pressure-cook chickpeas, water, kombu, and bay leaves for 2 hours. They should be very soft. (If boiling, please refer to Basic Bean Cooking Chart on page 98 for directions.)

While chickpeas are cooking, bring millet, water, and sea salt to boil in a medium-sized saucepan. Lower heat, cover, and simmer for 30 minutes. Set aside.

After chickpeas are completely cooked, remove bay leaves and drain, reserving bean liquid for soup stock. Mash kombu and half of the chickpeas with potato masher or fork. Stir mashed beans, carrot, onion, scallion, and tamari into hot, drained beans. Combine hot

---

*Lemon juice not recommended on a strict macrobiotic diet.

millet with chickpea mixture. Form into thin patties and pan-fry or bake on a lightly oiled baking sheet until crispy on the outside. If baking, use a 350°F oven for 20–30 minutes.

Purée sauce ingredients in a suribachi and serve over patties.

Alfredo Sauce

YIELD: ABOUT 2 CUPS

1 cup cannelloni beans (cooked or canned)
3 large cloves garlic
1 teaspoon Herbamare
¼ teaspoon nutmeg
8 ounces soy milk

You can either cook cannelloni beans as you would kidney beans (see chart on page 98) or use canned beans. Combine ingredients in a pan and cook on medium heat for 10 minutes. Pour contents into a blender and blend at a medium speed for about 3 minutes. Check for any lumps; gently stir and blend for a couple more minutes. Consistency should be fairly thick. Serve over your favorite pasta.

Enchiladas

YIELD: 12 ENCHILADAS OR 4 SERVINGS

Bean Filling
2 cups uncooked pinto beans
1 piece kombu, 6 inches long
6 cups water

1 bay leaf
¼ teaspoon sea salt

Sauce
3 tablespoons whole-wheat pastry flour
3 cups water or bean stock
1½ tablespoons tamari
1½ tablespoons umeboshi plum paste
1 teaspoon coriander
½ teaspoon ground cumin
½ teaspoon dry mustard
1–2 teaspoons cayenne
¼ teaspoon garlic powder
1 medium onion, chopped

Basic Enchiladas
¼ cup corn or safflower oil
12 corn tortillas (page 62)

Topping
12 green olives, sliced
3 scallions, sliced
1 recipe tofu cream dressing (page 20)

Pressure-cook beans, kombu, water, and bay leaf in a 4-quart or larger pressure cooker for 1 hour. (For boiling directions instead of pressure-cooking, please refer to Basic Bean Cooking Chart on page 98). Drain cooked beans and reserve bean stock. Pour beans and kombu back into pot, removing bay leaf. Add sea salt, and mash beans with a potato masher. Set aside, near stove.

Prepare sauce by combining all the sauce ingredients in a medium-sized saucepan, making sure flour is thoroughly dissolved. Stir over medium flame for 5–10 minutes until sauce thickens.

Heat oil in a frying pan large enough to hold an open tortilla. Using tongs, dip tortilla into oil for about 30 seconds, or until it becomes soft and pliable. Dip tortilla into sauce and

---

*Not recommended on a strict macrobiotic diet.

place it on a dinner plate or baking pan. Spread 1–2 tablespoons of mashed beans in a strip down the center of the tortilla. Fold each plain side of tortilla over filling, completely encasing bean mixture. Transfer bean enchilada to a 9- × 13-inch baking sheet and repeat process until all tortillas have been used up.

Pour remaining sauce over enchiladas. Sprinkle with olives and scallions, and bake at 350°F for about 15 minutes, or until hot. While baking, prepare tofu cream. Serve hot enchiladas garnished with tofu cream.

Imagination Lentil Burgers

YIELD: 4–6 SERVINGS

> 1 cup uncooked lentils
> 3 cups water
> 1 piece kombu, 4 inches long
> Cooked rice
> Toasted rye, barley, or oat flakes
> Parsley
> Onion
> Celery
> Miso
> Ground bay leaf
> Garlic

Pressure-cook lentils, water, and kombu for 30 minutes. (To boil, please refer to Basic Bean Cooking Chart on page 98 for directions.) Cooked lentils should be very soft. Be creative and combine cooked lentils with as much of the listed ingredients as needed to form a thick consistency. Form into burgers about 1-inch thick.

Place burgers on an oiled baking sheet and bake at 350°F for 30 minutes or to taste. The outside will be very crusty while the inside may be moist or dry, depending on the amount of liquid and other ingredients used. This dish is always interesting because it never comes out the same. Serve plain or with the sauce from the Crusty Millet Pizza With Carrot Sauce recipe on pages 74–75, or the sauce from the Lasagna on pages 81–82.

Lasagna Spirals

YIELD: 4–6 SERVINGS

Filling
1 cup uncooked chickpeas
4 cups water
1 piece kombu, 4 inches long
1 bay leaf
1 cup thinly sliced leeks
¼ cup chopped parsley
1 tablespoon light miso
*2 tablespoons lemon juice

Basic Lasagna
6 whole-wheat or artichoke lasagna noodles

Sauce
2 tablespoons grated carrot
1 tablespoon toasted sesame seeds (See page 30 for seed-toasting
*   directions.)*
¼ teaspoon grated ginger
1 cup water
2 teaspoons tamari
2 teaspoons kuzu

Pressure-cook chickpeas, water, kombu, and bay leaf for 2 hours or until soft. (If boiling, please refer to Basic Bean Cooking Chart on page 98 for directions.) While chickpeas are cooking, steam leeks for 2 minutes and set aside. As soon as chickpeas are cooked, remove bay leaf and discard. Remove chickpeas from their cooking liquid using a slotted spoon. Reserve cooking liquid. Purée chickpeas, kombu, steamed leeks, parsley, and miso in a food mill.

---

*Not recommended on a strict macrobiotic diet.

Add a little chickpea liquid if mixture is too dry to purée. The result should be the consistency of a thick spread. Stir in lemon juice.

Boil lasagna noodles for 15 minutes or until tender; drain, and rinse. Spread some of the chickpea mixture over each noodle, covering it completely. Roll the width of the noodle in jelly-roll fashion so you wind up with a chickpea-filled lasagna spiral. The filling will serve as a paste, enabling the noodle to hold its spiral shape. (Leftover spread may be used on sandwiches or crackers.)

In a large frying pan, combine sauce ingredients, thoroughly dissolving kuzu. Stir over medium heat for about 5 minutes until thickened and clear. Add spirals to pan and spoon a little sauce over each one. Heat over low flame until spirals are hot. If desired, use a carrot flower with an olive center to garnish each one. Serve hot or cold.

Leeks with Miso

by Julia Ferre
George Ohsawa Macrobiotic Foundation

YIELD: ABOUT 4 CUPS

1 medium bunch leeks
2 teaspoons light or dark sesame oil
2 teaspoons hatcho miso

Divide leeks into whites and greens by cutting at point where color changes. Remove roots and all outer inedible stalks. Slit whites in half lengthwise and open. Clean leeks by immersing them in a basin of cool water, thoroughly removing all sand from individual stalks. Rinse again, if necessary. Cut leek greens across into ½-inch pieces. Cut leek whites into ½-inch half rounds. Keep separate.

Heat oil in heavy pan over medium heat. Add leek greens and sauté until bright green, 1 to 2 minutes. Add leek whites and sauté 1 minute. Cover pan. Simmer over low heat for 7 to 10 minutes, until leeks have softened. Leeks will simmer in their own liquid. Add miso by spooning it on top of leeks. Cover pan and cook 1 to 2 minutes to soften miso. Gently stir miso into leeks until uniformly mixed and fragrant.

Colorful Luncheon Loaf

by Jackie Pukel
Oak Feed Natural Food Market and Restaurant

YIELD: 4–6 SERVINGS

1 large head of broccoli, sliced into chunks
1 medium buttercup squash, peeled and sliced into chunks
6 tablespoons whole-wheat flour
2 cups cooked millet (about 1 cup uncooked)

Steam broccoli and squash separately. Purée each of them in blender, food processor, or food mill. Add 3 tablespoons flour to each of the puréed vegetables. You should now have 3 distinct colors—green (broccoli), orange (squash), and yellow (millet).

Preheat oven to 350°F. Lightly oil a loaf pan. On the bottom, evenly spread out squash. Top with puréed broccoli, and top that with millet. Press millet down with your hands or a wooden spoon.

Bake for 30–40 minutes. Set loaf aside to cool for 30 minutes before turning upside down onto a serving platter. Slice and serve.

Sandy and Jackie Pukel

Oak Feed Natural Food Market and Restaurant
Coconut Grove, Florida

Sandy and Jackie Pukel are the founders of South Florida's most complete macrobiotic store, the Oak Feed National Food Market and Restaurant. Open since 1970, Oak Feed carries a variety of macrobiotic foods, as well as the most hard-to-find natural specialty foods available.

Buckwheat Cabbage Rolls

YIELD: 4 SERVINGS

Basic Cabbage Rolls
12 large cabbage leaves
1 cup uncooked buckwheat groats
2 cups water
Pinch sea salt
½ teaspoon coriander
2 tablespoons currants or raisins
1 cup chopped celery
½ cup sauerkraut, chopped
¼ cup toasted sunflower seeds (See page 30 for seed-toasting directions.)

Sauce
1 cup water
2 teaspoons kuzu
½ cup sliced leeks
1 tablespoon mirin
1 tablespoon tamari

Steam cabbage leaves until soft. Set aside to cool

Bring buckwheat groats, water, and sea salt to boil in a medium-sized saucepan. Lower heat, cover, and simmer for 20 minutes until buckwheat is cooked. Combine cooked buckwheat, coriander, currants, celery, sauerkraut, and seeds. Fill each cabbage leaf with about 2 tablespoons of buckwheat mixture and roll over, folding in the sides also. (See recipe for Egg Rolls on pages 116–117 and roll cabbage leaves the same way.) Secure each one with a toothpick and set aside.

Combine water, kuzu, leeks, mirin, and tamari in large saucepan, completely dissolving kuzu. Stir over medium heat until sauce is clear and leeks are cooked—about 5 minutes. Add cabbage rolls to simmering sauce and spoon sauce over each one. Heat rolls for about 10 minutes, and serve.

Variations

- Garnish with grated ginger.
- See recipes for Crusty Millet Pizza with Carrot Sauce on pages 74–75, Lasagna on pages 81–82, and Muffin Pizza on pages 84–85 for sauce recipes to use in place of kuzu-tamari sauce suggested here.

Sweet Stuffed Onions

YIELD: 6 SERVINGS

Basic Stuffed Onions
6 large onions
1 cup uncooked millet
2½ cups water
4 shiitake mushrooms
½ teaspoon sea salt
1 medium butternut, acorn, or buttercup squash cut into small chunks—about 4 cups peeled and cubed uncooked squash
6 springs parsley
*6 lemon slices

Sauce
1 cup water
1 tablespoon kuzu
1 tablespoon tamari

Peel onions. Place on a steaming rack in a large saucepan, bring about 2 inches of water to boil in the saucepan and steam whole, peeled onions for 10 minutes. Drain and set aside to cool.

---

*Not recommended on a strict macrobiotic diet.

Bring millet, water, shiitake mushrooms, sea salt, and squash to boil in a medium-sized saucepan. Reduce heat, cover, and simmer for 30 minutes. Remove shiitake mushrooms, chop, and return them to millet mixture, discarding tough stems. Stir grain, mashing some of the squash as you stir. Hollow out each onion with a spoon, leaving a ½-inch shell. Chop pulp and stir 1 cup of steamed onion pulp into millet stuffing. The rest of the onion may be used for soups, bean spreads, or whatever your imagination suggests. Fill each onion shell with millet stuffing. Place 6 onions in an 8- or 9-inch square or round baking dish with about ¼ inch of water on the bottom.

Prepare sauce by dissolving kuzu in water in small saucepan. Add tamari and stir over medium heat until sauce is thickened and clear. Spoon a tablespoonful of sauce over each onion. Place stuffed onions in 400°F oven for 15 minutes or until hot. Garnish each onion with a sprig of parsley and a lemon slice.

STEAMING VEGETABLES

Steaming permits vegetables to retain their moisture, sweetness, and nutritional value without the use of oil. This chart is composed of a list of vegetables for regular use that may be steamed. Though not intended to be an exhaustive list of vegetable choices, it does include some of the most often used vegetables on the macrobiotic diet.

To steam vegetables, a stainless-steel expandable steamer may be inserted into a two- or three-quart saucepan; a bamboo steamer may be used on top of a wok; or a specially made pot with holes on the bottom may be inserted into the appropriate-size saucepan.

To steam, bring a small amount of water to boil. Place the vegetables in the steamer, which is then inserted into or placed on top of the pot of boiling water, depending on which type of steamer you are using. Cover and cook over a medium-high flame for the length of time necessary to produce the desired softness. The longer the vegetables are steamed, the softer they will become. Check the water often so that it doesn't evaporate before the end of the cooking time. Leftover water may be saved for vegetable stock.

Vegetable Steaming Chart

Vegetable*	Amount of Water	Approximate Time	Results
2 cups acorn squash, cut into 1-inch chunks	2 cups	20 minutes	Soft
2 cups sliced bok choy, cut into 1-inch slices	¾ cup	3 minutes	Bright green leaves, crunchy stems
2 cups broccoli, cut into 1-inch chunks	¾ cup	5 minutes	Crunchy and bright green
2 cups brussels sprouts, halved	1½ cups	12 minutes	Soft and bright green
2 cups burdock, cut into ⅛-inch diagonal slices	1½ cups	10 minutes	Soft
2 cups buttercup squash, cut into 1-inch chunks	2 cups	20 minutes	Soft
2 cups butternut squash, cut into 1-inch chunks	2 cups	20 minutes	Soft
2 cups carrots, cut into ¼-inch diagonal slices	2 cups	15 minutes	Soft
2 cups carrot tops, chopped	¾ cup	3 minutes	Soft and bright green
2 cups cauliflower, cut into small flowerets	1½ cups	10 minutes	Soft, but not mushy
2 cups Chinese cabbage, cut into 1-inch slices	¾ cup	5 minutes	Mostly soft—thicker parts more crunchy
2 cups collard greens, cut into ½-inch slices	¾ cup	5 minutes	Semisoft, chewy, bright green

Vegetable*	Amount of Water	Approximate Time	Results
2 cups daikon, cut into ¼-inch diagonal slices	2 cups	15 minutes	Soft
2 cups green cabbage, cut into ½-inch slices	¾ cup	5 minutes	Slightly crunchy and bright green
2 cups kale, cut into 1-inch slices	¾ cup	5 minutes	Soft and bright, dark green
2 cups leeks, cut into 1-inch slices	¾ cup	5 minutes	Soft and bright green
2 cups onions, cut into quarters (small onions)	1½ cups	10 minutes	Soft
2 cups parsnips, cut into ¼-inch diagonal slices	2 cups	15 minutes	Soft
2 cups red radishes, halved	2 cups	15 minutes	Soft
2 cups rutabaga, cut into 1-inch cubes	2 cups	15 minutes	Soft
2 cups turnips, cut into ¼-inch slices	2 cups	15 minutes	Soft
2 cups turnip greens, cut into 1-inch slices	½ cup	3 minutes	Soft and bright green
2 cups watercress, cut into 1-inch pieces	½ cup	2 minutes	Soft and bright green

*Cut vegetables into bite-sized chunks or slices. If vegetables are not organically grown, as a general rule it is best to peel them. It is often preferable to peel organically grown vegetables as well, as sometimes the skins are bitter. If you choose to peel, the following vegetables are appropriate for peeling: all squashes, broccoli stems, carrots, daikon, parsnips, rutabaga, and turnips.

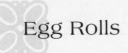
Egg Rolls

YIELD: 12 SMALL EGG ROLLS OR 4 SERVINGS

Basic Egg Rolls
2 teaspoons dark sesame oil
2 cups thinly shredded cabbage, Chinese cabbage, or bok choy
*½ cup diced green pepper
12 snow peas, sliced
2 cups mung bean sprouts
¼ teaspoon garlic powder
¼ teaspoon coriander
¼ teaspoon dry mustard
¼ teaspoon sea salt
12 egg roll wrappers
1 tablespoon arrowroot, diluted in 1 tablespoon water
¼ cup light sesame oil for frying

Apricot Sweet-and-Sour Sauce
½ cup dried apricots
½ cup water
¼ cup rice syrup
1 umeboshi plum, pit removed
¼ teaspoon dry mustard

Mustard Sauce
2 tablespoons dry mustard
3 tablespoons water

Heat dark sesame oil in a medium-sized frying pan or wok. Stir-fry cabbage, green pepper, snow peas, and sprouts for about 3 minutes, adding seasonings as they cook. Set aside to cool. Wrap all egg rolls as illustrated on next page and set aside onto a platter.

---

*Not recommended on a strict macrobiotic diet.

1. Place 1 tablespoon of filling on wrapper.

2. Fold pointed end over filling.

3. Fold in both side corners to completely cover filling.

4. Moisten flap with arrowroot mixture and roll over to seal.

Heat ¼ cup oil in saucepan until hot. Make sure egg rolls are dry before placing them in oil to eliminate excessive splattering. Place a few egg rolls in the oil at one time, and turn frequently with tongs or chopsticks until all sides are light golden brown. Transfer rolls to 9- × 13-inch baking sheet and place in 350°F oven to keep warm until ready to serve (no longer than 45 minutes, or they may get too dry).

While egg rolls are in oven, prepare apricot sweet-and-sour sauce by combining all sauce ingredients in a small saucepan and simmering for about 15 minutes. Purée sauce in a blender or food processor, adding more water if necessary to achieve desired consistency. Pour into a small bowl for serving.

To prepare dry mustard sauce, stir mustard and water together in a small bowl.

Serve egg rolls hot, with apricot sweet-and-sour sauce and dry mustard sauce on the side.

Variation

• Add small cubes of cooked seitan, tofu, or tempeh to the filling.

Millet "Mashed Potato" Pancakes

YIELD: 4–6 SERVINGS

2 cups millet
1 medium cauliflower, broken into about 4 cups of small flowerets
1 medium onion, chopped
5 cups water
¼ teaspoon sea salt
Light or dark sesame oil for oiling baking pans
1 recipe tofu cream dressing (See recipe on page 20 or use commercially
*   prepared soy or tofu sour cream.)*

Bring millet, cauliflowerets, onion, water, and sea salt to boil in a medium-sized sauce-pan. Lower heat, cover, and simmer for 30 minutes. While millet is simmering, prepare tofu cream and refrigerate it until serving time.

Purée cooked millet mixture in a food mill placed over a large mixing bowl. Form millet mixture into patties, using about 2 tablespoons of mixture for each pancake. Place them on 2 oiled 9- × 13-inch baking sheets. Broil pancakes 3–4 inches from flame, about 8 minutes on each side. You may also pan-fry instead of broiling. Remove from baking sheets and place on a platter. Serve garnished with 1 tablespoon of tofu cream on each one.

Quick Dumpling Sauté

by North Star Macrobiotic Center

YIELD: 4–6 SERVINGS

1 teaspoon light or dark sesame oil
2 medium onions, thinly sliced
1 medium daikon, thinly sliced

2 shiitake mushrooms, soaked and sliced
1 cup soft greens, such as mustard, Chinese cabbage, or napa, thinly sliced
2 slices whole-wheat bread
1 tablespoon shoyu

Brush oil in large frying pan and place on medium flame. When oil is hot, add onions and cook for one minute. Then stir in, one after the other, daikon, shiitake, the stems of the greens, and finally the bread. Add 3 tablespoons of water and cook for 30 minutes covered. Add extra water when necessary to prevent burning. Add the tops of the greens and shoyu without stirring them in. Cook 3 minutes more. Stir before serving.

Burdock-Onion Croquettes

by Jackie Pukel
Oak Feed National Food Market and Restaurant

YIELD: ABOUT 4 SERVINGS

Croquettes
1 cup grated burdock
1 cup grated onion
½ teaspoon sea salt
½–1 cup whole-wheat flour
light or dark sesame oil for deep-frying

Dip
¼ cup water
¼ cup tamari
½ teaspoon grated ginger

Combine grated burdock and onion in a medium-sized mixing bowl. Stir in sea salt and enough whole-wheat flour to bind vegetables together. Form into walnut-sized patties, balls, or oval shapes. Deep-fry in oil until golden brown.

Combine water, tamari, and grated ginger. Serve as a dip sauce with croquettes.

Summer Sea Palm

by The Mendocino Sea Vegetable Company

YIELD: 4–6 SERVINGS

2 cups dried sea palm fronds, packed
1–2 tablespoons olive oil
3 cloves garlic, crushed
*1 cup diced sweet red bell pepper
*1 cup diced green pepper
1 onion, diced
Sea salt or shoyu to taste

Soak sea palm in 4 cups warm water for 30 minutes. Drain, reserving water, and cut into 3-inch pieces. (For a dramatic effect, leave fronds full length.)

Heat 1 tablespoon oil in a wok or skillet, add sea palm and garlic, and sauté briefly. Cover and let cook for 20–30 minutes, adding soaking water as necessary to keep vegetables moist and to prevent sticking. (Use leftover water as a soup stock). Add pepper and onion and cook for 5 minutes more, adding 1 tablespoon more oil if desired, and soaking water as necessary. Season with sea salt or shoyu. Serve over rice or as a vegetable side dish. This versatile combination can also create cool summer salads when added to chopped lettuce or cooled rice.

---

*Not recommended on a strict macrobiotic diet.

The Mendocino Sea Vegetable Company

Mendocino, California

Eleanor Lewallen founded the Mendocino Sea Vegetable Company in 1980. She and her husband, John, wrote *The Sea Vegetable Gourmet Cookbook and Wildcrafter's Guide.* The Mendocino Sea Vegetable Company is committed to preventing drilling off the California coast, establishing a marine sanctuary, and harvesting and selling sea vegetables. You can find out more at www.seaweed.net.

Burdock, Carrot, and Lotus Root Kimpira

by Charles Gary and Mary David

YIELD: 4 SERVINGS

1½ tablespoons light or dark sesame oil
1 cup burdock, cut into thin slivers
Pinch sea salt
½ cup lotus root, cut into half-moons
½ cup carrots, peeled and cut into thin slivers
Water to cover
2 tablespoons shoyu

Heat oil in heavy skillet. Add burdock and sauté until strong scent is gone. Add pinch of sea salt and lotus root and carrot, and continue to sauté for 3–4 minutes. Add water to cover vegetables. Cover pan and simmer for 30–60 minutes until vegetables are very soft. Uncover, add shoyu, and cook until dry.

Ginger-Corn Dish

by Mary Wynne

YIELD: 4 SERVINGS

1 package dried tofu,
6 ears corn, shaved
1 tablespoon tamari diluted with 1 tablespoon water
½ package ginger pickles
*2 red bell peppers, diced

Rinse dried tofu and soak in water to cover until tofu expands. Squeeze water out of tofu, and cut into matchstick lengths.

Put ⅛ inch water into a large frying pan and heat. Add corn and cook for a few minutes. Place tofu on top of corn. Add diluted tamari to tofu. Cover, bring to boil, and lower flame to simmer for 10 minutes.

Add ginger pickles and simmer for about 3 more minutes. Add peppers and cook for 1 more minute. Remove from heat and serve.

Wakame, Squash, and a Crunch

YIELD: 4 SERVINGS

3 pieces wakame, 6 inches long
1 medium buttercup squash, peeled and cubed (about 4 cups of
cubed squash)
1 large onion, sliced

---

*Not recommended on a strict macrobiotic diet.

Water to cover
1–2 teaspoons tamari
1 tablespoon tahini
¼ cup toasted sunflower seeds (See page 30 for seed-toasting
  directions.)

Rinse wakame and soak in water for 5 minutes to soften. Slice each wakame piece lengthwise on either side of stem and discard stem. Slice stemless wakame pieces crosswise into squares or rectangles.

Place wakame, squash, and onion in a pot with water to cover. Bring to boil. Cover pot, lower heat, and simmer for 30–40 minutes. There should be very little or no water left by end of cooking time. If there is a lot of water left, cover and simmer a little longer, or drain off liquid and reserve it for soup stock. Add tamari and tahini toward the end of the cooking time. Stir all together so that squash falls apart and mixture becomes partly creamy.

Stir in seeds just before serving, and serve warm or at room temperature.

Navarro Oysters (Nori Tempura)

by The Mendocino Sea Vegetable Company

Yield: 4–8 servings

⅔ cup water
2 teaspoons kuzu powder
2 teaspoons natural soy sauce
Hot sauce or hot oil to taste
½ cup whole-wheat flour
1–2 tablespoons sesame seeds (optional)
1 egg (optional)
½ ounce dried nori
1 medium onion, diced
2 medium carrots or 1 yam, or both, peeled and cut into small pieces
½ cup safflower or light sesame oil

Combine ¼ cup water with kuzu powder and stir thoroughly to make a smooth paste. Then add the rest of the water. Add soy sauce and hot sauce or hot oil to taste. Combine this mixture with flour and sesame seeds to make a thin pancake batter. Stir in beaten egg, if desired. (Add more flour if you want to increase amount of batter.)

Break nori into small pieces or cut sheet nori into squares. Stir nori pieces into batter (The nori will absorb moisture in the batter.) Add onion and carrots or yam, or both.

To fry, pick up small amounts with chopsticks or a fork. Fry a few pieces at a time in hot oil until they are just beyond golden brown, and crisp on both sides. Remove, drain, and serve immediately as an appetizer (serves 8) or as a main dish (serves 4).

7.

❖ ❖ ❖

Fish

Fresh fish fits today's trend toward lighter, more nutritious, easily prepared foods. Fish is an excellent source of protein, vitamins, and minerals. It is especially high in vitamin B_{12}, which is a very difficult vitamin to get from a dairy-free, meat-free diet. Fish and shellfish may be seen as macrobiotic "fast food." They are easy and quick to prepare and delicious to eat.

Fish may be used in appetizers, spreads, dips, soups, salads, sauces, and main courses. It can be baked, broiled, fried, poached, steamed, boiled, and barbequed.

White-fleshed fish is the lowest in fat and can be eaten often. The varieties available include haddock, tilapia, cod, scrod, and flounder. Dark-fleshed, more oily varieties include salmon, bluefish, trout, mackerel, and sardines. Shellfish varieties include shrimp, scallops, clams, oysters, lobster, and crab. Garnish your fish with raw grated daikon or lemon, because they aid in digestion of the fish oils and help to emulsify them in the digestive process. Note: In recent years, mercury toxicity from eating certain types of fish has come into the public awareness. To maximize your vitality and health, it is best to limit or eliminate your intake of halibut, fresh tuna, swordfish, Chilean sea bass, and grouper.

Try to buy fresh fish the day you serve it. Make sure it is wrapped well and stored in the coldest section of your refrigerator until cooking time. If truly fresh, it should have no fishy odor.

When eating seafood in a restaurant, or serving it at home, try to include a variety of vegetable-quality foods such as raw or cooked salad, whole grains or pasta, and steamed or sautéed vegetables. These help balance out your meal.

Enjoy the recipes in this section, and use them as suggestions and ideas to help you create your own fish recipes.

Tangy Mustard Salmon

YIELD: 6 SERVINGS

1 tablespoon olive oil
3 tablespoons water
4 tablespoons prepared mustard
¼ medium onion, finely chopped
*1 tablespoon lemon juice
Pinch cayenne pepper
Any light oil for oiling broiling pan
6 salmon fillets, about ½ inch thick

Combine all ingredients except salmon. Preheat broiler. Lightly oil a broiling pan large enough to hold all the fish. Place fish on oiled pan. Spoon mustard sauce over salmon. Broil about 5 inches from heat for about 10 minutes or until fish tests done and topping is evenly browned. Thicker fish will take longer to cook. Serve garnished with lemon wedges and fresh parsley.

---

*Not recommended on a strict macrobiotic diet.

Garlic-Miso Monkfish

YIELD: 4 SERVINGS

> ¼ cup white miso
> 1 tablespoon rice syrup
> *1 tablespoon lemon juice
> 1 clove garlic, pressed or finely minced
> *1 pound monkfish, about ¾–1½-inch thick
> *Lemon slices

Combine miso with rice syrup, lemon juice, and garlic. Spread both sides of fish with this mixture, cover, and refrigerate for 24 hours.

To cook, place fish on rack in broiling pan (do not remove miso mixture). Broil 5–7 inches from heat for about 5 minutes on each side, depending on thickness of fish. Serve with lemon slices.

Mandarin Fish Broil

YIELD: 4–6 SERVINGS

> ⅓ cup tamari
> 1 tablespoon sesame oil
> 2 tablespoons water
> ¼ cup white wine
> ¼ medium onion
> 1 thin slice fresh ginger
> 1–2 cloves garlic

*Not recommended on a strict macrobiotic diet.

*1 tablespoon lemon juice
⅛ teaspoon cayenne (optional)
2 pounds haddock, scrod, or cod, ½ inch thick
Any light oil for oiling broiling pan
*Lemon wedges

Combine all ingredients except fish in a blender or food processor and blend until smooth. Pour the tamari mixture into a large bowl. Place pieces of fish into bowl and marinate in refrigerator for 30–60 minutes.

Preheat broiler. Place marinated fish on a lightly oiled broiling pan. Broil for about 8 minutes, about 5 inches from heat, or until fish flakes easily with a fork. Thicker fish will take longer to cook.

Garnish with lemon wedges.

Fillet of Sole Pinwheels

YIELD: 4–6 SERVINGS

¼ cup chopped almonds
2 cups whole-wheat cracker crumbs (I prefer a cracker made with oil, because it makes a richer-tasting stuffing.)
1 stalk celery
½ medium onion
⅛ teaspoon sage
½–¾ cup water
Any light oil for oiling baking pan
6 sole fillets, 6–8 inches long and ¼ inch thick
Parsley
Lemon wedges

Preheat oven to 375°F. With a wooden spoon, stir almonds in a small frying pan over medium flame until they are a light tan color. Place in medium-sized mixing bowl.

*Not recommended on a strict macrobiotic diet.

Blend several crackers in blender or food processor until fine. Continue until you have 2 cups. Add to almonds.

Dice celery and onions and add to crumb mixture along with sage and water. Stir well to combine ingredients.

Lay each piece of fish on a flat surface. Evenly divide stuffing into 6 portions and press each portion along the surface of each piece of fish. Roll each piece in a jelly-roll fashion and secure with a toothpick. Oil a medium-sized baking pan and place pinwheels on pan.

Cover fish with foil and bake for 20 minutes. Remove foil and continue baking for another 5–10 minutes until the center of each pinwheel flakes easily.

Garnish with sprigs of fresh parsley and lemon wedges.

Batter-Dipped Scrod

YIELD: 4 SERVINGS

Batter
½ cup cornmeal
½ cup rice flour
½ teaspoon sea salt
1 teaspoon mirin
1 cup water

Fish
1 pound scrod, cut into pieces about 2 x 3 inches
Safflower or light sesame oil for frying

Tartar Sauce
*¾ cup mayonnaise
*1 teaspoon lemon juice
½ teaspoon prepared mustard
1 tablespoon chopped dill pickle

---

*Not recommended on a strict macrobiotic diet.

Garnish
1 lemon, sliced in wedges

Combine batter ingredients in a medium-sized mixing bowl. Place fish on paper towels to remove excess moisture. Heat about ½ inch oil in a medium-sized frying pan. Dip each piece of fish into batter and place into hot oil. Fry for 4–5 minutes or until golden brown. Turn each piece with a spatula, and fry the other side. Remove fish from oil and place on plate covered with paper towels or a paper bag to absorb excess oil.

Combine tarter sauce ingredients in small bowl.

Serve hot fish with tartar sauce and lemon wedges on the side.

Pasta with Shrimp Sauce

YIELD: 4–6 SERVINGS

1 pound fresh shrimp (about 30–32 medium-sized shrimp)
Pinch sea salt
2 cloves garlic, minced
1 medium onion, chopped
*1 green pepper, diced
8–10 mushrooms, sliced
1 teaspoon sea salt
3 tablespoons olive oil
¼ cup water
1 pound udon, whole-wheat, or artichoke noodles
¼ cup chopped parsley
*1 lemon, sliced in 8 wedges

Purchase fresh, raw shrimp with heads removed. For each one, remove tail and peel. Make a slit down the back with a sharp knife, and remove vein. Fill a 2-quart or larger

---

*Not recommended on a strict macrobiotic diet.

saucepan halfway with water and a pinch of salt. Bring to boil over high flame and add shrimp. Boil shrimp for 2–3 minutes after water resumes boiling. Drain in a strainer and rinse under cold water to stop cooking process. Cut each shrimp in thirds and set aside.

If cleaned, boiled shrimp are purchased, eliminate shrimp cooking process and cut each one in thirds.

Sauté garlic, onion, green pepper, mushrooms, and salt in oil in a medium-sized saucepan for about 3 minutes. Add water and sauté for 5 more minutes or until vegetables are tender. Turn off flame. Cover and set aside.

Boil noodles for 10 minutes or until tender, and drain.

Add shrimp to vegetables and heat over medium flame until sauce is hot. Combine pasta and shrimp sauce in a large serving bowl. Sprinkle chopped parsley over the top, decorate with lemon wedges, and serve.

Marinated Fish Broil

YIELD: 4 SERVINGS

2–3 tablespoons tamari
1 tablespoon mirin
1 large or 2 small cloves garlic, minced
*Juice of ¼ lemon
1 pound scrod, haddock, or halibut
2 tablespoons toasted sesame seeds (See page 30 for seed-toasting
   directions.)

Combine tamari, mirin, garlic, and lemon juice in a 9-inch round or square baking pan. Add fish, turning it in marinade to evenly distribute seasonings. Marinate for 45–60 minutes. Remove fish from marinade and broil on a baking pan or on a rack placed inside a baking pan. Baste with more marinade, if desired, as fish cooks. Broil about 5–7 inches from flame for about 4 minutes on each side—longer for thicker fish. When done, sprinkle fish with toasted sesame seeds and serve.

---

*Not recommended on a strict macrobiotic diet.

Summer Somen with Fish

YIELD: 4 SERVINGS

1 cup water
¼ cup mirin
¼ cup tamari
1 teaspoon rice syrup
1 teaspoon grated ginger
1 pound white-fleshed fish
⅓ large, thin-skinned, burpless cucumber
1 pound somen noodles
16 snow peas
¼ cup toasted cashews or almonds (See page 30 for nut-toasting directions.)
3 scallions, finely chopped
4 sheets toasted nori, cut into strips

To make sauce, combine water, mirin, tamari, rice syrup, and grated ginger in small saucepan. Bring to boil and lower heat. Simmer for 5 minutes. Chill.

Cut fish into cubes and boil in salted water for about 3 minutes or until cooked through. Drain and chill.

Thinly slice cucumber, and set aside.

Boil somen for 7–8 minutes. Drain and set aside.

Steam snow peas until they are bright green and set aside.

Divide cooked somen into 4 bowls. Garnish each with fish, cucumber, snow peas, cashews or almonds, scallions, and nori strips. Divide sauce into 4 small bowls, so that each person has somen and garnishes.

8.

Salads, Pickles, Dressings, and Spreads

Fresh, raw vegetables with a tangy dressing, pasta dressed with a tahini sauce, or chilled boiled vegetables topped with creamy spiced tofu—salads of all types may be enjoyed on the macrobiotic diet. A hearty salad can be served with bread as a main course or a light salad can be served to add a delicate, special touch to your meal. A homemade salad dressing can enhance the flavor of any salad.

Pickled vegetables are often served in small amounts to add a salty, zesty taste to a meal and to aid digestion.

Bean and vegetable spreads on whole-grain bread or crackers come in handy for appetizers, sandwiches, and snacks. They are a quick refreshing way to eat beans, vegetables, and grains.

Avocado Macaroni Salad

YIELD: 4 SERVINGS

Dressing
½ small onion, diced
*2 tablespoons lemon juice
4 tablespoons light sesame oil
½ teaspoon prepared mustard
½ teaspoon sea salt

Basic Salad
1 cup uncooked artichoke or whole-wheat macaroni
1 medium carrot, diced
1 celery stalk, diced
1 small avocado
¼ cup chopped parsley
1 scallion, chopped
¼ cup toasted sunflower seeds (See page 30 for seed-toasting directions.)
4 large or 8 small green olives, sliced

Purée onion, lemon juice, oil, water, mustard, and salt in blender, food processor, or suribachi. Set aside.

Boil macaroni in a medium-sized saucepan for 10–15 minutes or until tender. Drain macaroni and place in medium-sized salad bowl. Set aside to cool.

Steam carrot and celery for 2 minutes until cooked but still firm. Slice avocado in half, remove pit, and peel. Cut into ½-inch chunks. Place steamed vegetables, avocado, parsley, scallion, sunflower seeds, and olives in salad bowl with macaroni. Moisten salad with as much dressing as desired, and mix well. Serve immediately, or refrigerate for 1 hour before serving.

---

*Not recommended on a strict macrobiotic diet.

Quick and Tasty Noodle-Vegetable Delight

by Meredith McCarty
author of *American Macrobiotic Cuisine*

YIELD: 3 SERVINGS AS A MAIN DISH

Vegetables
2 quarts (8 cups) water
1 medium onion (or equivalent amount of leeks, halved lengthwise to clean between leaves, or green onions), thinly sliced
1 medium carrot, peeled and halved lengthwise, each half thinly cut into diagonals
4 cups broccoli, tops separated into flowerets, tough bottom portion discarded, stems sliced into thin diagonals

Noodles
8 ounces whole-grain noodles, any kind

Dressing
2 tablespoons dark sesame oil or olive oil
3–4 tablespoons good quality soy sauce or umeboshi vinegar to taste

Bring water to boil in a large saucepan while you cut vegetables. Add all vegetables and cook until just tender, about 5–8 minutes. Drain, returning broth to pot for cooking noodles.

Cook noodles until done (tender but firm), about 8–12 minutes, depending on the kind. Drain and run them under cool water to prevent sticking, if not serving immediately.

Prepare dressing by combining ingredients. Mix noodles or pasta with vegetables and pour dressing over gradually for strength desired.

Variation

- Use other green vegetables in place of broccoli such as: brussels sprouts, bok choy, cabbage, kale, watercress, or big sprouts such as sunflower, mung, or soybean. Boil softer greens for only 2 minutes before adding them to salad.

Chickpea Salad with Sesame-Lemon Dressing

by Margaret Lawson
founder and director of the Macrobiotic Center of Dallas

YIELD: 4 SERVINGS

2 cloves garlic, minced
¼ cup toasted sesame seeds
½ teaspoon sea salt
*¼ cup fresh lemon juice
¼ cup extra-virgin olive oil
1 zucchini squash (cut in matchsticks)
2 carrots (cut in matchsticks)
2 cup chickpeas, cooked and drained
¼ cup parsley (washed, drained and chopped)
¼ cup scallions (thinly sliced)

Dressing: Process garlic, toasted sesame seeds, and salt in food processor. While food processor is running, add lemon juice and oil and blend until smooth. Set aside.

Salad: Quick boil zucchini in boiling water until just tender, about 5 seconds. Remove and drain. Quick boil carrots matchsticks in the same boiling water about 2 to 3 minutes. Remove and drain. Toss together carrots, zucchini, chickpeas, and dressing in a large mixing bowl. Stir in parsley and scallions and toss to coat with dressing.

NOTE: This dish keeps in refrigerator two or three days and is a hit at potluck dinners.

---

*Not recommended on a strict macrobiotic diet.

Margaret Lawson

Founder and director of the Macrobiotic Center of Dallas

In addition to her work at the Macrobiotic Center of Dallas, Margaret has owned and operated two restaurants in Dallas—the Macro Gourmet and the Macro Café—as well as a macrobiotic cooking school. She currently teaches cooking classes on a regular basis and will be opening a macrobiotic bed-and-breakfast in the fall of 2003.

Lentil and Orzo Salad

by Margaret Lawson

YIELD: 4 SERVINGS

1 cup organic green lentils
1 cup orzo pasta (or other small pasta)
½ cup Natural Italian Salad Dressing
1 tablespoon Dijon mustard
½ cup celery, cut in thin slices
2 carrots, cut in thin matchsticks

Cook lentils until just tender (but not mushy), about 10 or 15 minutes. Cook orzo or other small pasta according to package directions; drain and set aside. In a small bowl, combine salad dressing and mustard. Set aside.

In a small saucepan, bring 2 cups water to a boil. Add carrots and cook about 2 minutes; remove and drain. Add celery and cook about 1 minute; remove and drain. In a large mixing bowl, combine cooked lentils, orzo, celery, and carrots. Stir in dressing and toss well.

Red Radish Pickles

by Aveline Kushi and Wendy Esko
Authors of *The Changing Seasons Macrobiotic Cookbook*

YIELD: 1 CUP PICKLES

1 cup sliced red radishes
2 umeboshi plums
Small amount sea salt

Place radishes in pickle press or small bowl. Break umeboshi apart and add to radishes. Sprinkle on a little sea salt, mix, and press. Leave for 3–4 hours. Remove and place on serving dish and serve.

Black and White Noodle Salad

YIELD: 4 SERVINGS

½ cup uncooked arame
1 large onion, sliced
Water to cover
1 cup cauliflowerets
1 cup uncooked whole-wheat or artichoke shells or macaroni
1 teaspoon tamari
1 teaspoon umeboshi vinegar
1 teaspoon mirin
2 scallions, chopped
Parsley sprigs

Soak arame in water to cover until soft. Drain, cut it into 1-inch pieces, and place in a 2-quart or larger saucepan. Add onion and water to cover. Bring arame mixture to boil. Lower heat, cover, and simmer for 45 minutes.

While arame is cooking, steam cauliflowerets for 5–8 minutes until they are soft, and set aside.

After 45 minutes, most of the arame water will have evaporated, but there should be about 1 inch left on the bottom. If there is too much or too little liquid, adjust it accordingly by boiling off some of the liquid or adding a little water. Add shells, tamari, umeboshi vinegar, and mirin. Simmer, covered, for 10 minutes or until shells are tender. Stir in steamed cauliflower and raw scallions. Let arame mixture rest in pot, covered, for 1 minute. This will slightly wilt the scallions so that they are not raw tasting. Remove ingredients from pot and set aside in a bowl to cool. Serve at room temperature, garnished with a sprig of parsley in the center.

Variation

• Add a handful of roasted almonds to the cooled salad mixture.

Arame Salad

YIELD: 4 SERVINGS

1 cup dry arame (soak in water to cover for about 10 minutes and drain the water)

1 medium carrot, cut into matchsticks

1 medium onion, sliced

Water to cover

¼ pound tofu, cut into small cubes

1 tablespoon dark sesame oil

1–2 teaspoons tamari

¼ teaspoon grated ginger

½ cup sauerkraut

2 tablespoons toasted sesame seeds (See page 30 for seed-toasting instructions.)

Bring arame, carrot, onion, and water to cover to boil in a medium-sized saucepan. Lower heat, cover and simmer for 45 minutes.

While arame is cooking, pan-fry tofu cubes in oil until they are lightly browned, and set aside.

When arame is cooked, add tamari and simmer a few minutes longer. There should be very little water left. Transfer hot arame to bowl and stir in tofu, ginger, sauerkraut, and sesame seeds. Cool to room temperature and serve.

The Community of Ionia, Alaska

The community of Ionia is a rural, family-oriented macrobiotic village of forty-five people living in self-built log cabins. We work together to maintain organic gardens, a grain field, a large log community center, a ball field, and a sledding hill. We have lots of wild land for our many growing children and new babies being born all the time (we are now third generation!).

Sea Palm Salad

by the Community of Ionia, Alaska

YIELD: 4–6 SERVINGS

Dressing
1 large or 2 small carrots, minced
½ cup dark sesame oil
1 cup mirin
*5 or 6 lemons, juiced
½ cup scallions, thinly sliced
Umeboshi to taste

**Not recommended on a strict macrobiotic diet.

Sauté minced carrot in dark sesame oil until soft and sweet. Add mirin and simmer for 3 minutes. Let cool. Place in suribachi or large bowl. Add lemon juice, scallions, and ume-boshi and shoyu to taste. Set aside.

Salad
4–5 handfuls sea palm
Shoyu to taste
2 English cucumbers
1 head red-leaf lettuce
½ cup red onions, minced

Rinse, then soak, 4 or 5 large handfuls of sea palm in pot. Boil about 15 minutes with shoyu and strain. Half-peel cucumbers and slice into diagonal half-moons. Clean and break lettuce. Mince red onion. Combine sea palm, cucumbers, lettuce, and onion in a large bowl. Toss with dressing and serve.

Carrot Salad

YIELD: 4 SERVINGS

Dressing
⅛ pound tofu
1 tablespoon light sesame oil
1 teaspoon rice vinegar
1 teaspoon rice syrup
⅛ teaspoon sea salt
3 tablespoons water

Basic Salad
3 medium carrots, peeled and grated
¼ cup raisins

Boil tofu for 1 minute and remove from water. Blend tofu, oil, rice vinegar, rice syrup, sea salt, and water in blender, food processor, or suribachi until smooth.

Combine carrots, raisins, and dressing. Refrigerate for at least 1 hour before serving.

Variations

- Use ½ cup commercially prepared soy or tofu mayonnaise or salad dressing instead of the recipe above.
- Add ¼ cup nuts or seeds to the basic salad.
- Add 2 tablespoons of grated coconut to the basic salad.

Squash Spread

by Susan Hamill

YIELD: 2–3 CUPS

2–3 cups peeled, cooked, and puréed winter squash (dry types are best,
    like Hokkaido and buttercup)
1½ tablespoons sweet white miso or light red miso
1½ tablespoons tahini
2 tablespoons finely chopped scallions

Combine all ingredients in a medium-sized bowl and mix well. Serve on rice, unleavened bread, or rice cakes. This makes an excellent snack, school lunch, or traveling food.

Sushi Salad

by The Mendocino Sea Vegetable Company

YIELD: 4–6 SERVINGS

1 tablespoon rice malt
1 tablespoon sesame seeds
8 cups cooked rice, cooled
3 tablespoons diced onion
4 tablespoons shoyu
1 teaspoon sesame oil (optional)
1 teaspoon grated fresh ginger
1 teaspoon rice vinegar
2 cups loosely packed roasted nori
1 cup parsley, chopped

Liquefy rice malt in small saucepan over low heat. (Don't add water to rice malt. It will thin over the low heat and will then easily mix into the rice.) Roast sesame seeds in dry skillet or pan over medium-low heat, stirring constantly until they smell fragrant and begin to pop.

In large bowl, combine all ingredients, adding nori and parsley last, and reserving ¼ cup of each for garnish.

Waldorf Salad Variation

YIELD: 4 SERVINGS

1 tablespoon white miso
¼ medium onion, chopped and steamed
*1 tablespoon lemon juice

---

*Not recommended on a strict macrobiotic diet.

2 tablespoons water

4 medium apples, cut into ½-inch chunks (Red delicious apples work well.)

2 celery stalks, cut into thin slices

¼ cup raisins

¼ cup toasted nuts or seeds (See page 30 for nut-toasting directions.)

Purée miso and steamed onion with lemon juice and water in a suribachi or blender. Drop apple chunks into boiling water for 30 seconds and remove. (They should still be firm, but not raw.) Do the same with the celery. Combine all ingredients and chill. This salad looks attractive served on a bed of lettuce.

Snow Peas and Cauliflower Salad

YIELD: 4 SERVINGS

Basic Salad

1 medium head cauliflower

1 cup snow peas

Dressing

2 tablespoons toasted sesame seeds (See page 30 for seed-toasting directions.)

2 tablespoons umeboshi plum paste

*2 tablespoons lemon juice

4 tablespoons water

1 scallion, sliced

---

*Not recommended on a strict macrobiotic diet.

Break cauliflower into small flowerets, lightly steam, and place in salad bowl. Flowerets should be cooked, but still firm. Steam snow peas for a few minutes until their color turns bright green, and combine them with cauliflowerets.

Combine sesame seeds, umeboshi plum paste, lemon juice, and water in a small bowl and mix well. Spoon as much of this dressing as you desire over steamed vegetables, and stir. Top with sliced, raw scallions. Serve cool or at room temperature.

Quinoa Salad with Tahini Dressing

by Margaret Lawson
founder and director of the Macrobiotic Center of Dallas

YIELD: 4 SERVINGS

Quinoa Salad
1 cup quinoa
1½ cup water
¼ teaspoon sea salt
½ cup carrots, finely cubed and quick boiled
6 scallions, thinly sliced
Parsley, washed, drained, and chopped
½ cup sliced almonds, toasted
Tahini Dressing (recipe follows)

Bring 1½ cups water to a boil, covered. Remove lid and add quinoa and sea salt. Cover and return to boil. Reduce heat and simmer 15 minutes. Turn flame off and allow to sit covered for 5 minutes. Remove cooked quinoa to a mixing bowl. Stir in cooked carrots, scallions, parsley, and toasted almonds. Serve on individual plates and drizzle Tahini Dressing over each serving.

Tahini Dressing
¼ cup raw tahini
2 garlic cloves, minced
1 or 2 tablespoons natural soy sauce

*¼ cup lemon juice
½ cup water

Combine all ingredients in a food processor and blend until creamy. Add a little more water, if needed, for thinner consistency.

Spring Salad

YIELD: 4 SERVINGS

Basic Salad
5 red radishes, sliced in rounds
1–2 scallions, finely chopped
1 head iceberg lettuce, thinly sliced
1 large celery stalk, thinly sliced
1 cucumber (peeled if waxed), thinly sliced

Dressing
1 small onion, diced
¼ pound tofu
1 tablespoon tahini
1 tablespoon dark miso
½ teaspoon prepared mustard
2 tablespoons water

Combine basic salad ingredients in a medium-sized salad bowl and refrigerate.

Boil diced onion in about ½ inch of water for 2–3 minutes or until pearly white, and place in small mixing bowl. Boil tofu for 1–2 minutes and place in the same mixing bowl, adding tahini, miso, prepared mustard, and water. Mash all dressing ingredients with a fork until they are thoroughly blended.

Stir tofu mixture into basic salad, mix well, and serve chilled.

---

*Not recommended on a strict macrobiotic diet.

Salad with Miso Dressing

YIELD: 4 SERVINGS

Dressing
1 small or ½ medium onion, sliced
2 tablespoons mellow barley miso
½ teaspoon dry mustard
2 tablespoons rice syrup
3 tablespoons light sesame oil
3 tablespoons rice vinegar

Basic Salad
8 asparagus spears, cut into 2-inch lengths
1 head leaf lettuce, torn into pieces
1 cup mung bean sprouts
½ cup grated carrots
¼–½ cup pitted black olives

Steam onion for 2 minutes or until soft. Purée onion with other dressing ingredients in blender, food processor, or suribachi until smooth. Set aside.

Steam asparagus for 3–5 minutes or until tender, and place in a medium-sized salad bowl. Add lettuce, sprouts, carrots, and olives. Toss salad with as much dressing as needed to coat vegetables. Serve at room temperature or chilled.

Leftover dressing can be stored for about 5 days if refrigerated.

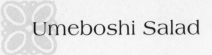

Umeboshi Salad

YIELD: 4 SERVINGS

Basic Salad
½ medium head cabbage, thinly sliced
1 celery stalk, thinly sliced
1 bunch watercress, chopped

Dressing
½ medium onion, diced and steamed for 1 minute
¼ teaspoon grated ginger
1 umeboshi plum (pit removed) or 1 teaspoon umeboshi plum paste
½ teaspoon dark sesame oil
¼–½ cup water

Drop cabbage into a pot of boiling water just until cabbage changes color. Remove from pot with slotted spoon and let cool in medium-sized bowl. Repeat this procedure with celery and watercress.

Purée dressing ingredients in a suribachi or blender. Add enough water to achieve a creamy consistency. Pour dressing over vegetables, toss, and serve.

Marinated Daikon-Carrot Salad

YIELD: 4 SERVINGS

> 1½ cups grated daikon
> 1½ cups grated carrot
> 1 tablespoon tamari
> ½ teaspoon dark sesame oil

Combine all ingredients and marinate in a cool place for 2–4 hours before serving.

Chilled Peppers and Tofu Salad

YIELD: 4 SERVINGS

> *3 red or green peppers
> ½ teaspoon dried basil
> 1 clove garlic, minced
> 1 tablespoon olive oil
> 5 scallions, cut into 1-inch lengths
> ½ pound firm tofu, cut into ½-inch cubes
> 2 teaspoons tamari
> ¼ cup water
> 1 tablespoon umeboshi vinegar

Slice peppers in rings and remove seeds. Slice each ring in half. Stir-fry basil, garlic, and peppers in olive oil in a medium-sized saucepan for 5 minutes. Add scallions, tofu, tamari, and water. Bring to boil, lower heat, and simmer for about 10 minutes until water is evaporated.

---

*Not recommended on a strict macrobiotic diet.

Add umeboshi vinegar and remove pan from heat. Refrigerate for at least 1 hour before serving to allow salad to marinate. Serve chilled.

Green Goddess Dressing

YIELD: ½–1 CUP DRESSING, DEPENDING ON AMOUNT OF WATER USED

1 medium onion, sliced
¼ cup water
3 umeboshi plums, pits removed
½ cup chopped parsley
2 scallions, chopped
½ cup cooked rice (pressed into measuring container)
¼ teaspoon tamari
1–2 tablespoons olive oil

Simmer onion in water covered for 3–5 minutes or until transparent. Purée all ingredients in a blender, adding a small amount of water if mixture appears to be too thick. Refrigerate and serve over vegetable, grain, noodle, or bean salads.

Dill Pickles

by Aveline Kushi and Wendy Esko
authors of *Changing Seasons Macrobiotic Cookbook*

YIELD: 2 POUNDS PICKLES

¼–⅓ cup sea salt
8–10 cups water
1 cup onions, sliced in thick half-moons

1–2 sprigs fresh or dried dill
1 cup carrots, sliced thinly on a diagonal
2 pounds fresh pickling cucumbers, quartered lengthwise

Place sea salt in a large pot, add water, and mix. Bring to boil. Reduce flame to medium and simmer about 5 minutes or until salt has dissolved. Remove from flame and allow to cool.

Place onions in a large (1-gallon) glass jar or crock and add about one quarter of the dill. Then, place carrot slices on top of onions and add a little more dill. Finally, place cucumber spears in jar or crock and add remaining dill. Pour cool salt water over vegetables. (If you use hot water, vegetables will not pickle properly and may become soft and mushy.) Cover top of jar with a piece of cheesecloth so that air can get at it.

Let vegetables sit in salt water for 3–4 days. Pickles ferment better if kept in a cool (not cold), dark place. When cucumbers change from bright green to a dull green color, cover jar and refrigerate 1–2 days longer. After 1–2 days refrigeration, pickles are ready to use. In the summer months, when the weather is very hot, these pickles may need to sit out in the open only 1–2 days before being refrigerated. If pickles are too salty for your liking, rinse under cold water. Serve in bowl or on pickle tray.

Rutabaga-Tamari Pickles

by Aveline Kushi and Wendy Esko
Changing Seasons Macrobiotic Cookbook

YIELD: 2 CUPS PICKLES

2 cups rutabaga, quartered or cut in eighths and thinly sliced
Water
Tamari

Place sliced rutabaga in pickle press, small ceramic crock, or bowl. Prepare a mixture of half water and half tamari, enough to cover rutabaga halfway. Put top on pickle press and screw down. If using a crock or bowl, place a plate and some kind of weight on top of the rutabaga. Leave 4 hours or overnight. These pickles will keep about 1 week. If they become too salty, simply wash or soak them to remove excess tamari before serving.

Wendy Esko

Clinton, Michigan

When Wendy began following the macrobiotic way of life in the early 1970s, she was unaware of the changes it would make in her life. As she became healthier and more balanced, her whole sense of life became one of challenge and excitement.

Through her many cooking classes and books, Wendy has been able to share her excitement, knowledge, and experience about macrobiotics. She has written *The Changing Seasons Macrobiotic Cookbook* (with Aveline Kushi); the recipe section of *The Macrobiotic Way;* and *The Macrobiotic Cancer Prevention Cookbook* (with Aveline Kushi).

Green Herbal Dressing

by Spring Street Natural Restaurant

YIELD: ABOUT 3 CUPS

*1 cup (tightly packed) fresh spinach leaves, rinsed and drained
1 cup (loosely packed) fresh parsley leaves
½ cup cider vinegar
1½ teaspoons dried basil, crumbled
1½ teaspoons sea salt
½ teaspoon freshly ground black pepper
½ teaspoon ground cumin
2 cloves garlic
1½ cups olive oil

*Not recommended on a strict macrobiotic diet.

Combine spinach leaves, parsley, vinegar, basil, sea salt, pepper, cumin, and garlic in a food processor; process until smooth. With machine running, slowly add ½ cup oil; add remaining oil all at once. Process until smooth. Store dressing in tightly covered container in refrigerator up to 3 weeks.

Macro-Style Barbecue Sauce

by Sprout House

YIELD: ABOUT 2 QUARTS

1 bottle Westbrae Tofu Sauce
½ cup tamari
4 cups spring water
1 cup barley malt
¼ cup toasted sesame seeds (See page 30 for seed-toasting directions.)
2 jars Soken Peanut Sauce

Combine all ingredients in a medium-sized bowl. Cover and let sauce rest in refrigerator for 2–3 days. This allows flavors to blend together. If too strong or salty, add more spring water. This sauce will last a whole summer if kept refrigerated.

Presteamed tempeh (20 minutes), tofu, seitan, fish, or vegetable chunks can be marinated in this mixture for 6–12 hours, or simply brushed with the sauce before grilling. Barbecue for 10–15 minutes (depending on what you are cooking), brushing with more sauce if desired.

Navy Bean Seed Spread

YIELD: ABOUT 2 CUPS OF SPREAD, OR 4 SERVINGS

1 cup uncooked navy beans
3 cups water
1 piece kombu, 4 inches long
½ medium onion, chopped
1 tablespoon miso
½ teaspoon crumbled dried dill or 1 teaspoon chopped fresh dill
2 tablespoons toasted sunflower or sesame seeds (See page 30 for seed-
    toasting directions.)
2 scallions, finely chopped

Pressure-cook navy beans, water, and kombu for 50 minutes. (If boiling, please refer to Basic Bean Cooking Chart on page 98 for directions.) Drain excess liquid from cooked beans through a strainer and into a bowl to be reserved for soup stock, and return beans to pressure cooker.

Stir onion, miso, and dill into beans and mash with a potato masher to achieve the consistency of a chunky spread. Stir in seeds and scallions. Let cool to room temperature before serving on bread, rice cakes, or crackers.

Miso-Lemon Bean Spread

YIELD: ABOUT 2 CUPS OF SPREAD, OR 4 SERVINGS

1 cup uncooked great white northern beans
3 cups water
1 piece kombu, 4 inches long

1 bay leaf
1 clove garlic
1 medium carrot, peeled and sliced
1 tablespoon miso
*2 tablespoons lemon juice

Pressure-cook beans, water, kombu, bay leaf, and garlic for 50–60 minutes. (If boiling, please refer to pinto bean recipe on Basic Bean Cooking Chart on page 98.)

While beans are cooking, steam carrot slices until very soft, and set aside.

The cooked beans should be very soft. Remove bay leaf from beans and discard. Transfer beans, kombu, garlic, carrot, miso, and lemon juice to a food mill. Purée bean mixture, adding a small amount of bean liquid if necessary. Reserve extra bean liquid to be used for soup stock. Bean mixture should be the consistency of a thick spread.

Serve warm or cool, on crackers or sandwiches, as a dip, or as a side dish.

Variations

- Add ¼ cup diced celery or scallions to the puréed bean mixture.
- Add ¼ cup finely chopped onion to the puréed bean mixture.

Tempeh-Olive Sandwich Filling

Yield: Filling for 4 sandwiches

8 ounces (1 package) tempeh, cut into 1-inch cubes
4-inch piece kombu, broken into small pieces
1 medium onion, chopped
Water to cover
1 tablespoon light miso
1 tablespoon lemon juice* or rice vinegar

*Not recommended on a strict macrobiotic diet.

1 tablespoon water
⅛ teaspoon grated ginger
1 tablespoon tahini
¼–½ cup diced celery
¼ cup sliced green or black olives

Place tempeh, kombu, and onion in a 2-quart or larger saucepan with water to cover. Bring to boil, lower heat, and simmer for 30 minutes. There should be almost no water remaining. Mash cooked tempeh with fork or potato masher. Combine with miso, lemon juice, water, ginger, tahini, celery, and olives. Stir to distribute seasonings evenly. Serve at room temperature or chilled, on sourdough whole-grain bread with mustard, if desired.

Garlic Tossed Salad

Yield 4 servings

Basic Salad
1 head romaine lettuce, torn into pieces
1 carrot, grated
1 scallion, sliced
1 cucumber, sliced
½ cup pitted black olives

Dressing
3 tablespoons olive oil
3 tablespoons umeboshi vinegar
½ teaspoon rice syrup
2 cloves garlic, minced
¼ teaspoon prepared mustard

Combine basic salad ingredients in a medium-sized mixing bowl. Combine dressing ingredients in a jar and shake well. Pour desired amount of dressing over salad, toss, and serve.

9.

❖ ❖ ❖

Desserts

Are you looking for low-fat, low-cholesterol, sugar-free, dairy-free desserts that are satisfying as well as nutritious? The recipes in this section are just what you are looking for!

As you begin to appreciate the flavor of whole foods, the natural sweetness of barley malt, rice syrup, maple syrup, and fruit-sweetened desserts will become increasingly more gratifying. Try experimenting with your favorite desserts to make them more nutritious. Refined sweeteners can be replaced with natural ones. Unrefined corn oil may be used in place of half or all the butter in a recipe. Whole-wheat pastry flour may be used in place of bleached white flour.

Eating healthfully doesn't have to mean giving up desserts; it can mean eating homemade treats prepared with natural ingredients and a caring touch.

Apple Strudel

YIELD: 1 STRUDEL OR 4 SERVINGS

Dough
1¼ cups whole-wheat pastry flour
¼ cup rice flour
⅛ teaspoon sea salt
¼ cup corn oil
¼ cup water

Filling
2 medium apples, peeled, cored, and sliced
½ cup raisins
½ cup water
1 teaspoon kuzu
Pinch sea salt
¾ cup chopped walnuts or pecans

To make dough, stir flours and sea salt together in a medium-sized mixing bowl. Add oil and water and stir until mixture is the consistency of soft dough—it doesn't take much stirring. With your hands, form dough into a ball and set aside. Do not knead.

In small saucepan, combine all filling ingredients except nuts, making sure kuzu is thoroughly dissolved. Stir over medium heat until filling mixture has become transparent and fruit is glazed with a thick, clear sauce. Let cool.

To assemble, roll out dough between 2 sheets of waxed paper. Roll as thin as possible without tearing dough. Remove top piece of waxed paper.

At this point, there are 2 styles of strudel to choose from.

Style 1: Spread cooled filling over rolled-out dough. Top with nuts. Fold edge of dough closest to you over about 2 inches of filling. Roll that part over the next 2 inches and keep rolling strudel in jelly-roll style until dough is used up. Place strudel on an oiled 9- × 13-inch baking sheet, and slice some diagonal slits on top of it using a sharp knife. Bake at 400°F for about 40 minutes or until golden brown.

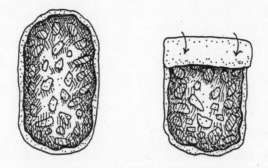

Figure 9.1

Style 2: Place rolled-out dough onto an oiled 9- × 13-inch baking sheet. Spread cooled filling in a wide strip down the center ⅓ of the dough. Sprinkle with nuts. Cut horizontal slits in sides of dough as pictured in Figure 9.2. Fold each piece of side dough over the center strip of filling to form a braid down the center as pictured in Figure 9.3. Bake at 400°F for 20–30 minutes or until golden brown.

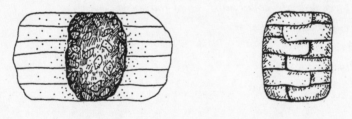

Figure 9.2   **Figure 9.3**

For both styles: Remove cooked strudel from pan and place on a rack to cool, or slice on baking sheet and place slices on a rack to cool. Serve warm or at room temperature.

Variations

- Use peaches, pears, blueberries, or cherries in place of apples.
- Drizzle ¼–½ cup barley malt, rice syrup, or maple syrup over cooked strudel and place under broiler for a few minutes to form a glaze.

Strawberry-Pear Pie

YIELD: 9-INCH PIE OR 4–6 SERVINGS

Crust
1 cup uncooked couscous
2 cups apple juice
pinch salt
1 tablespoon toasted sunflower seeds (See page 30 for seed-toasting directions.)
2 tablespoons fruit-juice-sweetened preserves

Filling
1 tablespoon kuzu, dissolved in ¾ cup apple juice
1 large pear or 2 small pears, cored and sliced
1 cup sliced strawberries
½ cup raisins
Pinch sea salt
1 tablespoon rice syrup

Bring couscous, apple juice, and salt to boil in a medium-sized saucepan. Lower heat and simmer for 5–7 minutes. Cover couscous mixture and set aside for about 5 minutes until all the liquid is absorbed. Stir in the sunflower seeds, and with moistened hands, press the couscous mixture into a 9-inch pie plate. Spoon the fruit-juice-sweetened preserves over the piecrust and place under a broiler for a few minutes until the preserves are bubbly. Remove from broiler and set aside ready to be filled.

Bring dissolved kuzu, apple juice, pear, strawberries, raisins, pinch sea salt, and rice syrup to boil in a 2-quart or larger saucepan. Lower heat and simmer for 10–15 minutes, stirring often, until pear slices are soft. Pour filling into prepared crust and chill for 1–2 hours before serving.

Variations

- Instead of strawberries, used pitted cherries, blueberries, or raspberries.
- Use the same crust and fill it with mashed yams or parsnips.

Couscous Apple Pie

YIELD: 9-INCH PIE OR 4–6 SERVINGS

Crust
1 cup uncooked couscous
2 cups apple juice
Pinch sea salt
2 tablespoons chopped nuts
2 tablespoons fruit juice-sweetened preserves

Filling
6 medium apples
1 tablespoon kuzu, dissolved in ¾ cup water
Pinch sea salt
½ teaspoon cinnamon
2 tablespoons raisins
¼ cup apple juice

Bring couscous, apple juice, and salt to boil in a medium-sized saucepan. Lower heat and simmer for 5–7 minutes. Cover couscous mixture and set aside for about 5 minutes until all the liquid is absorbed. Stir in nuts, and with moistened hands, press the couscous mixture into a 9-inch pie plate. Spoon the fruit-juice-sweetened preserves over the piecrust and place under a broiler for a few minutes until the preserves are bubbly. Remove from broiler and set aside ready to be filled.

Slice apples or cut them into ½-inch chunks. Peel them if desired. Place apples in a 2-quart or larger saucepan with dissolved kuzu liquid, pinch sea salt, cinnamon, raisins, and apple juice. Bring apple mixture to boil, lower heat, and simmer for 10–15 minutes, stirring often, until apples are soft. Pour filling into prepared pie shell, and let cool. Refrigerate for 1–2 hours before serving. Serve cool or at room temperature.

Mochazake Pie

by Jessica Porter

Yield: 8 servings

Pie Crust
1½ cups whole-wheat pastry flour
¼ teaspoon sea salt
¼ cup safflower oil
¼ cup cold apple juice

Preheat oven to 375°F. Combine flour, salt, and oil together, mashing with a fork. When mixed together, slowly add the apple juice to create a dough. Knead the ball of dough for a few minutes. Roll the dough between two sheets of wax paper, making a circle approximately 10 inches in diameter. Lay the circle in a prepared 9-inch pie tin. Prick the dough liberally with a fork. Cover the pie tin with aluminum foil, laying it right against the dough and folding it over the sides of the crust. Bake for 15 minutes. Remove foil and bake for 5 more minutes. Set aside to cool.

Filling
1 quart of plain amazake (set aside ¼ cup for diluting kuzu)
*½ cup hazelnut butter
2 tablespoons grain coffee
1 teaspoon umeboshi vinegar

---

*Feel free to adjust the nut butter and grain coffee ratios to strike your personal fancy. You can also experiment with different crusts or serve this dish simply as a pudding.

½ teaspoon vanilla (optional)
3 level tablespoons agar-agar flakes
2 tablespoons kuzu

Blend amazake, hazelnut butter, grain coffee, vinegar, and vanilla in a blender until smooth. Pour into a saucepan, stir in agar-agar, and bring to boil over a medium flame. Reduce the flame to low and let simmer 15 minutes, whisking regularly to prevent sticking and also to help the agar-agar dissolve. Be sure to cook it the full 15 minutes, even if it appears that the agar-agar has dissolved, to avoid lumps after setting.

Dilute kuzu in ¼ cup cold amazake and add to pot. Stir constantly to avoid lumps. Bring to a boil again, then back to a simmer. After about a minute, the mixture should thicken slightly. Pour into prepared piecrust and let set. Garnish with crushed roasted hazelnuts and a light sprinkling of grain coffee.

Strawberry Cream Pie

by Eric Stapelman
The Macrobiotic Center of New York

YIELD: 1 10-INCH PIE

CRUST
Dry Ingredients
½ cup almond flour (ground almonds)
½ cup oat flour (ground oats)
½ cup whole-wheat flour
Pinch sea salt

Wet Ingredients
*¼ cup maple syrup
¼ cup corn oil
½ teaspoon vanilla extract

---

*Not recommended on a strict macrobiotic diet.

Mix wet ingredients and dry ingredients separately and then add them together. Press onto a lightly oiled 10-inch pie pan, making sure to press evenly. Bake for 20–25 minutes at 350°F or until golden—not brown.

Filling
1 quart apple-strawberry juice
1½ pints fresh strawberries
6 ounces rice syrup
1½ level teaspoons agar flakes
½ teaspoon vanilla extract
3 tablespoons arrowroot powder

Blend juice, fruit, and rice syrup. Put in a medium-sized pot and add agar. Bring to boil slowly and whisk continuously. Boil for just 3 minutes. Add vanilla extract.

Dilute arrowroot in 4 tablespoons cold water and whisk into fruit mixture. Pour into prebaked pie crust and let cool. Garnish with fresh berries.

Eric Stapelman

The Macrobiotic Center of New York
New York, New York

Throughout Eric's many years of teaching and cooking professionally, he has found that dessert recipes are the ones that people remember him for. Eric hopes that many people will enjoy this recipe and his recipe for Almond Raspberry Cake on page 182.

Apple-Raisin Butter

YIELD: 1–1½ CUPS

1 cup apple juice
1½ cups raisins
Pinch sea salt

Combine all ingredients in a medium-sized saucepan. Bring to boil. Lower heat, and simmer for 15–20 minutes. Purée in blender, food processor, or food mill until smooth.

Variations

- Add ¼ cup chopped nuts to the puréed mixture.
- Use 1 cup of orange juice* in place of apple juice.
- Add ¼–½ teaspoon cinnamon to puréed mixture.

Apple Dumplings

YIELD: 4 DUMPLINGS

Pastry
2 cups whole-wheat pastry flour
¼ cup + 2 tablespoons corn oil
½ teaspoon sea salt
¼ cup + 3 tablespoons water

---

*Not recommended on a strict macrobiotic diet.

Filling

4 medium apples, peeled and cored (MacIntosh work well)

4 pinches sea salt

4 tablespoons apple butter

4 teaspoons raisins

Sauce

1 tablespoon kuzu

1 cup water

Pinch sea salt

*¼ cup maple syrup

½ cup toasted chopped walnuts (See page 30 for nut-toasting
*   directions.)*

Preheat oven to 400°F. Combine pastry flour, oil, and sea salt in a medium-sized mixing bowl, stirring with whisk or wooden spoon to make sure ingredients are evenly distributed. Stir in water until dough can be shaped into a ball. Usually ¼ cup plus 3 tablespoons water is sufficient, but sometimes different flours absorb water differently, and a little more water may be needed to form a soft dough that can be rolled out. Press and knead dough into 2 balls.

Roll out each ball of dough between 2 pieces of waxed paper. Try to form dough into a rectangular shape. Cut each rectangle in half.

Place an apple on top of each piece of dough, and put a pinch of sea salt inside each apple. Spoon 1 level tablespoon of apple butter and 1 teaspoon of raisins inside the core of each apple. Fold opposite ends of dough over each apple and press ends of dough firmly, completely covering the whole apple and sealing in filling. With sharp knife, make slits in the dough at the top of each apple to allow steam to escape. Transfer uncooked dumplings to a 9-inch square or larger baking dish. Bake for 50–55 minutes.

While dumplings are baking, prepare sauce. Dissolve kuzu in water in small saucepan. Add sea salt, maple syrup, and walnuts, and stir over medium heat for about 5 minutes, or until thickened. Serve warm sauce over slightly warm or room-temperature dumplings.

---

*Not recommended on a strict macrobiotic diet.

Almond Orange Cookies

YIELD: 14 COOKIES

1 cup almonds
1 cup whole-wheat pastry flour
⅛ teaspoon sea salt
½ cup raisins
*¾ cup orange marmalade (Sorrel Ridge is good)
*2 tablespoons maple syrup
¼ cup corn oil
½ teaspoon vanilla

Finely grind almonds in food processor or blender. Combine ground almonds with remaining ingredients, and mix well.

Form walnut-sized balls of cookie dough and place on an oiled 9- × 13-inch baking pan. Press each cookie with a fork to flatten to about ¼-inch thick. Bake at 400°F for 20 minutes. Remove from pan with a spatula and place on a wire rack to cool.

Award-Winning Strawberry Pie

by Meredith McCarty
author of *American Macrobiotic Cuisine*

YIELD: 1 PIE

Basic Single-Crust Pie Dough
⅓–½ cup water or apple juice
1½ tablespoons corn oil

---

*Not recommended on a strict macrobiotic diet.

¼ teaspoon sea salt
1½ cups whole-wheat flour (bread and/or pastry)

Filling
3 pints strawberries
½ teaspoon sea salt
½ cup brown rice syrup
½ cup agar flakes
1 sprig fresh mint for garnish (optional)

Preheat oven to 350°F. To prepare Basic Single Crust Pie Dough, heat water, oil, and sea salt to lukewarm in a medium-sized saucepan. (Volume of liquid varies, depending on texture of flour). This thoroughly dissolves the salt and makes for a smoother dough. Add warmed liquid to flour in a medium-sized mixing bowl. Stir to form a kneadable dough, then knead quickly to make dough smooth, soft, and easy to work with. Add more flour only if necessary. Roll dough out immediately, as an all-whole-wheat-pastry flour dough tends to harden with time. Transfer to lightly oiled pie pan. Crimp edges and bake until edges are barely golden, about 15 minutes. Allow crust to cool slightly before filling. (Roll out any extra dough for crackers by sprinkling seeds, crushed nuts, herbs, or other seasonings on the surface before rolling. Cut with knife, pastry wheel, or cookie cutters and bake as for pie crust.)

To prepare filling, rinse strawberries in a saucepan by placing them in a bowl of cool water and rinsing them quickly. Pinch off stems after rinsing so none of the flavorful juice is lost in the water. Place whole strawberries in medium-sized saucepan and sprinkle with salt. Pour rice syrup over berries and sprinkle agar flakes over all. Cover pan and bring to boil, then simmer until agar is completely dissolved, about 15 minutes. Strawberries are so full of liquid (about ½ cup comes out) that no liquid is necessary as long as you keep heat at medium-low. Stir several times.

Pour filling into prebaked crusts. Allow to jell, about 3 hours at room temperature or 2 hours in a cooler place. To garnish pie, place fresh mint sprig in center of the pie after it has partially jelled.

Pecan Oatmeal Cookies

YIELD: 15–18 COOKIES

> ½ cup corn oil
> 1 cup barley malt
> 1 teaspoon vanilla
> ¼ teaspoon sea salt
> 1 cup whole-wheat pastry flour
> ½ cup water
> 2 cups uncooked rolled oats
> ½ cup chopped pecans

Combine all ingredients in large mixing bowl. Drop by teaspoonfuls onto an oiled cookie sheet. Flatten each cookie with a fork. Bake in 350°F oven about 30 minutes, or until golden brown.

Rich and Creamy Squash Pie

YIELD: ONE 9-INCH PIE OR 4–6 SERVINGS

Couscous Crust *(page 161)*

Filling
1 medium buttercup squash, peeled and cubed (about 4 cups of cubed squash)
2 cups amasake
1 cup roasted and peeled fresh chestnuts or ¾ cup dried chestnuts (soaked overnight in water to cover)
⅛ teaspoon sea salt
1 teaspoon cinnamon

½ teaspoon almond extract
1 tablespoon kuzu, dissolved in ¼ cup water

Topping
½ cup Crispy Brown Rice (Can be purchased in natural foods store.)
2 tablespoons barley malt

Prepare couscous crust to fit 9-inch pie pan using either the recipe on page 160 or the recipe on page 161. Set aside and prepare filling.

Pressure-cook squash, amasake, chestnuts, and sea salt for 30 minutes. Purée this mixture in a food mill, blender, or food processor, adding cinnamon and almond extract. Transfer squash purée to a 2-quart or larger saucepan.

Add dissolved kuzu to squash purée and stir over medium heat for 5–10 minutes or until mixture thickens—it should have the consistency of thick pudding. Pour this filling into couscous pie shell and let cool.

Sprinkle Crispy Brown Rice over cooled filling. Heat barley malt in small saucepan over medium heat for 2–3 minutes until thin. Drizzle warm barley malt over Crispy Brown Rice and put pie under broiler for 1–2 minutes to glaze. Serve at room temperature.

Variation

- Use ½ cup of granola for topping in place of Crispy Brown Rice.

Holiday Pudding

by Mary Wynne

YIELD: 6 SERVINGS

Pudding
¾ cup couscous
4–5 cups apple or peach juice
1 cup water
2 cups cooked sweet rice
½ cup raisins

¼–½ cup tahini or almond butter
¼–½ cup barley malt
2 tablespoons vanilla
¼ teaspoon sea salt

Fruit Glaze
4 cups apple juice or peach juice
1 pound cranberries (wash and remove bad berries)
½ teaspoon sea salt
*1–3 tablespoons maple syrup
3 tablespoons kuzu
½ cup water

Combine all pudding ingredients in a 4-quart or larger pressure cooker. Cook for 15 minutes after pressure comes up. Let cooked pudding cool in pressure cooker.

Heat apple or peach juice for glaze in large saucepan. Add berries, sea salt, and maple syrup. Simmer for 5–10 minutes. Dissolve kuzu in ½ cup water and stir it into glaze mixture for thickening.

Spoon pudding into dessert cups. Top with fruit glaze. Cool or refrigerate to set before serving.

ABC Pudding

Yield: 6–8 servings

2 cups uncooked whole-wheat alphabet noodles
4 medium apples, peeled, cored, and thinly sliced
¼ cup raisins
¼ cup barley malt
⅛ teaspoon sea salt

---

*Not recommended on a strict macrobiotic diet.

2 tablespoons arrowroot

Water

1 cup toasted, chopped almonds, pecans, or walnuts (see page 30 for
nut-toasting directions.)

In a medium-sized saucepan, combine uncooked noodles, apples, raisins, barley malt, salt, and arrowroot. Add just enough water to cover, and make sure arrowroot is completely dissolved before heating. Bring to boil, lower heat, and simmer over medium heat for about 15 minutes, adding ½ cup more water if liquid gets too thick or evaporates too much. Stir a few times to keep noodles from sticking to bottom of pot. After 15 minutes, mixture should be the consistency of thick oatmeal with most of the water absorbed.

Stir in nuts and press mixture into a lightly oiled 8- or 9-inch round or square baking pan. Bake uncovered at 350°F for 20 minutes. Cool pudding and slice into squares before serving.

Strawberry-Apple Parfait

YIELD: 4 SERVINGS

1½ cups uncooked short-grain brown rice

2¼ cups water

Pinch sea salt

2 tablespoons kuzu, dissolved in 1 cup water

⅛ teaspoon sea salt

2 cups applesauce

2 cups sliced strawberries

¼ cup rice syrup

2 tablespoons tahini

1½ cups toasted pecans, almonds, or walnuts, chopped (See page 30
for nut-toasting directions.)

Pressure-cook rice, water, and pinch sea salt for 45 minutes. (If boiling, please refer to Basic Grain Cooking Chart on page 50 for directions.)

Place dissolved kuzu, sea salt, applesauce, strawberries, rice syrup, and tahini in a 2-quart or larger saucepan. Bring fruit mixture to boil, lower heat, and simmer for 10 minutes, stirring often. Mixture should thicken. Remove from heat and stir in 3 cups of cooked rice. Layer pink rice mixture in parfait glasses. Alternate layers of mixture with layers of nuts. Top with sprinkling of nuts. Refrigerate and serve chilled.

Apple-Glazed Tropical Couscous

YIELD: 4 SERVINGS

Couscous Pudding
1½ cup uncooked couscous
½ cup raisins
½ cup coconut, grated
½ cup toasted almonds, chopped (See page 30 for nut-toasting directions.)
1 cup amasake
2½ cups water
¼ teaspoon sea salt

Glaze
1 tablespoon kuzu
1 cup apple juice
Pinch sea salt

To make couscous pudding, bring all ingredients to boil in a medium-sized saucepan. Lower heat and simmer over low flame for about 10 minutes. Water should be absorbed into pudding and each grain of couscous should be soft and puffed. (If at the time the water is absorbed, the grain does not look this way, add a little more water and simmer until the couscous is soft.) Press mixture firmly into an 8-inch round or square pan or into 4 individual dessert dishes. Set aside to cool.

Make glaze in a small saucepan. Dissolve kuzu in apple juice with a pinch of salt added. Stir over medium flame until juice thickens. Spoon over couscous and spread evenly. A glazed appearance and texture will be formed as it cools.

Nutty Sweet Fruit Supreme

YIELD: 4 SERVINGS

½ cup dried apricots
½ cup raisins
Water
4 medium pears, peeled, cored, and sliced
4 medium apples, peeled, cored, and sliced
1 cup raw pecans or almonds
Pinch sea salt

Soak apricots and raisins in water to cover for at least 30 minutes. Combine all ingredients, including water from soaking the apricots and raisins, and bake in a covered 8-inch baking dish at 350°F for 40 minutes. Stir occasionally while baking. Uncover and bake 10 more minutes to form a slight crust on top. Serve warm or cool.

Variations

- Add spices such as ¼ teaspoon cinnamon, ¼ teaspoon coriander, or ¼ teaspoon cardamom.
- Add a vanilla bean and remove after baking.

Oatmeal Cookies

by Jackie Pukel
Oak Feed Store

YIELD: ABOUT 2 DOZEN COOKIES

3 cups whole-wheat flour
1½ cups rolled oats
1 cup chopped almonds
Pinch sea salt
1 cup raisins (optional)
¼ cup corn oil
½–1 cup rice syrup or barley malt (depending on desired sweetness)
1 tablespoon vanilla
1 cup water

Preheat oven to 350°F. Mix dry ingredients together in large mixing bowl. Stir wet ingredients together and add them to dry. Add more water if batter is too dry. With a wet tablespoon, spoon dough onto an oiled cookie sheet. Press down with fork. Bake for 25–30 minutes.

Crispy Rice Balls

YIELD: 6–8 RICE BALLS

2 cups crispy brown rice cereal
¼ cup almond butter
2 tablespoons crushed walnuts
¼ cup rice syrup
2 tablespoons grain-sweetened chocolate chips

Combine all ingredients thoroughly in a large mixing bowl. Taking a heaping teaspoon of the rice mixture into your moistened hands, form the rice into a small ball, pressing the ingredients together. Continue this process until all the ingredients are used up, moistening your hands with water between the making of each ball. Store in a sealed container or plastic bag in the freezer or refrigerator.

Variations

* Use peanut or cashew butter or seseame tahini instead of almond butter.
* Use ½ cup instead of ¼ cup rice syrup for a sweeter flavor.
* Replace the walnuts with almond, peanuts, or cashews.

Almond-Butter Oatmeal Cookies

YIELD: 12 COOKIES

1¼ cups uncooked rolled oats
½ cup rice flour
2 tablespoons corn oil
⅛ teaspoon sea salt
⅓ cup raisins
¾ cup apple juice
¼ cup toasted almond butter
½ teaspoon vanilla
*½ cup shredded coconut
*3 tablespoons maple syrup

Preheat oven to 400°F. Combine all ingredients in a large mixing bowl and stir well. Drop by spoonfuls onto an oiled 9- × 13-inch baking sheet. Flatten each cookie with fork to

*Not recommended on a strict macrobiotic diet.

about ¼-inch thick. Bake for 30 minutes or until golden brown. Remove from pan and place on a wire rack to cool.

Carob Brownies

Yield: 12 small brownies

¼ cup raisins
1¼ cups whole-wheat pastry flour
¼ cup soy flour
¾ cup rice syrup
½ cup roasted carob powder
½ cup chopped walnuts or pecans
1 teaspoon vanilla
¼ teaspoon sea salt
¼ cup corn oil
¾–1 cup water

Stir all ingredients together in medium-sized mixing bowl, adding water to achieve a thick, brownie-batter–like consistency. Bake in an oiled 8-inch square baking pan for about 60 minutes at 350°F or until a toothpick comes out clean when poked into brownies. Let brownies cool before slicing.

Variation

- For a lighter consistency, add 1 beaten egg to the batter.

Squash-Chestnut Pudding

YIELD: 4 SERVINGS

1 cup dried chestnuts, soaked in water to cover overnight
1 medium buttercup squash, peeled and cubed (about 4 cups of
*   cubed squash)*
2 cups apple juice
½ teaspoon cinnamon
⅛ teaspoon sea salt
½ cup toasted almonds (see page 30 for nut-toasting directions.)
2 tablespoons barley malt
*2 tablespoons maple syrup
¼ teaspoon vanilla

Pressure-cook chestnuts, squash, apple juice, cinnamon, and sea salt for 30 minutes. Purée chestnut mixture in food mill, blender, or food processor until smooth. Transfer purée to an 8-inch round or square baking dish. Chop toasted almonds and sprinkle them on top of pudding. Stir barley malt, maple syrup, and vanilla together in small bowl and drizzle over chopped almonds. Place pudding in broiler for about 3 minutes, or until almonds are glazed with barley malt and vanilla. Serve warm or cool.

Nutty Apricot Pastries

YIELD: 16 PASTRIES

2 cups whole-wheat pastry flour
¼ teaspoon sea salt
⅓ cup corn oil

---

*Not recommended on a strict macrobiotic diet.

¼ cup water
¾ cup apricot preserves or jam
½ cup raisins
½ cup chopped walnuts
2 teaspoons cinnamon

Combine flour, salt, oil, and water in a large mixing bowl. Stir with a whisk or wooden spoon to evenly distribute oil throughout the flour. Mold dough into 2 balls with your hands, adding 1–2 tablespoons more water if dough is too dry to mold.

Between 2 sheets of waxed paper, roll 1 ball of dough into 9-inch circle. Remove top sheet. Spread entire circle with half of the preserves, sprinkle with half of the raisins, half of the nuts, and 1 teaspoon of cinnamon. Cut circle into 8 pie-shaped wedges. From the wide end of each wedge, roll each piece of dough, pressing the point of the wedge against the rolled pastry to keep it from unraveling. Place each pastry on an oiled 9- × 13-inch baking pan. Repeat this process with the other ball of dough and remaining filling ingredients.

Bake at 350°F for 25–30 minutes.

Please note: The preserves may run, so please remove pastries from baking pan and place onto cooling rack as soon as they are taken out of oven. If this is not done, and the preserves have run, pastries may stick to baking pan and will be more difficult to remove later.

Pecan Rush

YIELD: 12 PASTRIES

Crumble Pastry
1½ cups of whole-wheat pastry flour
¼ teaspoon sea salt
⅓ cup corn oil
¼ cup water

Filling

1 cup raw pecans

1 beaten egg (preferably from a free-running hen fed organic feed)

⅛ teaspoon sea salt

½ cup rice syrup

¼ teaspoon vanilla

2 tablespoons water

Topping

*¼ cup maple syrup

Preheat oven to 400°F. Combine all pastry ingredients in medium-sized mixing bowl with wooden spoon or whisk. Make sure oil is evenly distributed throughout flour. With your hands, crumble flour mixture into well-oiled 9-inch round or square baking pan and set aside.

Finely grind pecans in blender or food grinder. Combine all filling ingredients in medium-sized mixing bowl, stir well, and spread filling evenly over pastry. Drizzle maple syrup over filling and bake for 30 minutes. Cool and cut into 12 pieces. Remove from baking pan if desired, and serve.

Raisin-Pecan Cookies

by Mary Wynne

YIELD: 4 DOZEN

3 cups rolled oats

2¼–2½ cups whole-wheat pastry flour (or sweet rice flour)

1 teaspoon sea salt

2 teaspoons baking soda

---

* Not recommended on a strict macrobiotic diet.

¼ cup chopped pecans

½–¾ cup raisins

½ teaspoon cinnamon

¾ cup corn oil

*1¼ cups maple syrup

¼ cup water

2 tablespoons rice vinegar

2 tablespoons vanilla

Combine oats, flour, sea salt, and baking soda in a bowl. Stir in nuts, raisins, and cinnamon. Add corn oil. Mix well to make sure oil coats all of the flour.

In separate bowl, combine maple syrup, water, vinegar, and vanilla. Add this wet mixture to dry ingredients and mix well.

Lightly oil cookie sheets and drop teaspoonfuls of cookie dough onto the sheets. Bake at 350°F for 15–17 minutes.

Almond-Butter Vanilla Bars

YIELD: ABOUT 16 BARS

Basic Bars

2 eggs (preferably from free-running hens fed organic feed)

½ cup corn oil

1 teaspoon vanilla

1 cup amasake

*½ cup maple syrup

½ teaspoon sea salt

3 cups whole-wheat pastry flour

1 tablespoon baking powder

⅓ cup raisins

---

* Not recommended on a strict macrobiotic diet.

Frosting
1 cup toasted almond butter
¼ teaspoon sea salt, if the almond butter is unsalted
½ cup rice syrup
3–4 tablespoons water to achieve a smooth spreading consistency

Beat eggs, oil, vanilla, amasake, maple syrup, and sea salt in medium-sized mixing bowl. Stir in flour, baking powder, and raisins. Pour batter into an oiled and floured 9- × 13-inch baking pan or into 2 oiled and floured 8-inch layer cake pans. Bake at 350°F for 20–25 minutes or until a toothpick comes out clean, and set on rack to cool.

To prepare frosting, combine almond butter, salt, rice syrup, and water and stir well. Spread frosting on cooled bars, slice, and serve.

Variations

- Substitute carob chips for raisins.
- Substitute currants for raisins.
- Mix ½ cup grated coconut into the batter or the frosting.

Almond Raspberry Cake

by Eric Stapelman
The Macrobiotic Center of New York

YIELD: 10-INCH CAKE

Dry Ingredients
2 cups almond flour
2 cups whole-wheat pastry flour
*2 cups unbleached white flour
3 tablespoons baking powder

---

*Not recommended on a strict macrobiotic diet.

Wet Ingredients
18 ounces soy milk
¾ cup corn oil
*¾ cup maple syrup
1½ cups apple juice
1 teaspoon almond extract
1 jar raspberry conserves

Garnish
Fresh raspberries
Toasted almonds, chopped

Mix dry ingredients and wet ingredients (except for raspberry conserves) separately in 2 large mixing bowls. Then, add wet ingredients to dry, leaving out raspberry conserves, and stir until combined—not too long. Pour ingredients into 2 lightly oiled 10-inch spring-form pans. Bake at 350°F, checking with a toothpick after 20–25 minutes.

Let cakes cool and remove them from pans. Spread tops of both with conserves, then place on top of the other. Garnish with fresh raspberries and chopped toasted almonds.

Please note that if cake rises too high in the center, you can cut top off to make it level.

Sunny Apple Spice Cake

by Sue Segal

YIELD: 12-INCH CAKE

5 cups diced, unpeeled apples
3 tablespoons cinnamon
1 tablespoon allspice
1 teaspoon cloves (optional)
3 cups whole-wheat pastry flour

---

*Not recommended on a strict macrobiotic diet

3 teaspoons baking powder
½ teaspoon sea salt
1 cup raisins (preferably golden)
¾ cup corn oil
1 cup barley malt
1½–2 cups water
Sunflower seeds or nuts

Combine apples with spices in a large bowl and let sit until spices have been absorbed into apples. Add flour, baking powder, sea salt, and raisins. Mix well, then add oil, barley malt, and water and combine. Batter will now be thick. Pour into an oiled and floured 12-inch springform pan. Top with raw sunflower seeds or nuts of your choice. Bake at 350°F for 45–60 minutes. This cake is moist and works best in the springform pan, so you don't have to transfer it to another plate to serve it.

Quick Poppy Seed Cake

by Jacqueline Wayne

YIELD: ONE 9- × 13-INCH CAKE, OR TWO 8-INCH ROUND CAKES

1½ cups barley malt
⅓ cup corn oil
¾ cup raisins
1 cup boiling water
4 cups whole-wheat pastry flour
1 teaspoon sea salt
1 teaspoon baking powder
1 cup poppy seeds
¼ teaspoon cinnamon
¼ teaspoon cloves
¾ cup chopped almonds

Combine barley malt, corn oil, and raisins in medium-sized mixing bowl. Pour boiling water over this and mix well. This procedure helps blend mixture more evenly into flour. Add flour, sea salt, baking powder, poppy seeds, cinnamon, and cloves. Stir just enough to moisten and blend. Pour into an oiled 9- × 13-inch baking dish or 2 round 8-inch cake tins. Sprinkle with chopped almonds. Bake at 375°F for 25–35 minutes, or until top springs back when lightly touched.

Apple Crunch Cake

YIELD: 4–6 SERVINGS

Bottom Layer
1 cup apple juice
¼ cup corn oil
¼ cup water
½ teaspoon vanilla
¼ teaspoon sea salt
1½ cups whole-wheat pastry flour
1 tablespoon baking powder

Middle Layer
4 medium MacIntosh apples
1 teaspoon cinnamon

Top Layer
¼ cup barley malt
¼ cup rice syrup
2 tablespoons corn oil
½ teaspoon vanilla
¼ teaspoon sea salt
1 cup uncooked rolled oats
1 cup chopped walnuts

To prepare bottom layer, combine apple juice, oil, water, vanilla, and sea salt in medium-sized mixing bowl. Add dry ingredients and mix only until combined. Pour mixture into an oiled and floured 9-inch round or square baking pan.

To prepare middle layer, peel, core, and thinly slice apples. Layer apple slices on top of batter and sprinkle with cinnamon.

To prepare top layer, heat barley malt, rice syrup, and oil in medium-sized saucepan over medium heat for 3–5 minutes, or until thin. Stir in rest of ingredients and crumble this mixture over the apple layer.

Bake at 350°F for 50 minutes. Slice and serve warm or cool.

Sticky Pecan Rolls

YIELD: 12–14 SMALL ROLLS

Basic Rolls
*1 tablespoon yeast, dissolved in ¼ cup water
1 cup water
¼ cup rice syrup
2 tablespoons corn oil
1 teaspoon sea salt
2 cups whole-wheat flour
1 cup unbleached white flour

Filling
1 teaspoon cinnamon
1 tablespoon corn oil
1 tablespoon rice syrup
½ cup chopped pecans

---

*Not recommended on a strict macrobiotic diet.

Topping
2 tablespoons corn oil
2 tablespoons rice syrup
*2 tablespoons maple syrup
1 tablespoon water
¼ cup chopped pecans
Pinch sea salt

Combine all basic roll ingredients and knead for 5 minutes or until smooth. Place dough in oiled medium-sized mixing bowl, cover with a clean towel, and let rise for 1–1½ hours. Punch down and roll out to a 12- × 14-inch rectangle.

Combine cinnamon, corn oil, and rice syrup in small saucepan. Stir over medium heat for a few minutes until rice syrup is thin and easily pourable. Spread cinnamon mixture over rolled-out dough and sprinkle with ½ cup chopped pecans. Roll up dough in jelly-roll fashion, pressing the open end against the roll in order to seal the open side. Set oven for 350°F.

Cut roll into 1-inch pieces. Place topping ingredients in a 9-inch baking pan. Place pecan roll pieces over the topping ingredients. Cover rolls with damp cloth and let rise until double. Bake at 375°F for about 30 minutes or until done. Remove from oven. Turn pan upside down onto serving platter and serve warm.

---

*Not recommended on a strict macrobiotic diet.

10.

❊ ❊ ❊

Beverages

Bancha tea, pure spring water, and grain coffee are the main beverages suggested on the macrobiotic diet. They are caffeine-free and contain no sugar, artificial coloring, preservatives, or other additives. Bancha tea, sometimes called kukicha, is a mild, balanced tea that is suitable for everyday use. Grain coffee is a caffeine-free coffee substitute made mostly from roasted grains that have been finely ground. Grain coffee may also be taken frequently.

Pure, unsweetened fruit juices may be used occasionally, but not in large quantities. I like to serve my children apple juice diluted with twice as much water as juice. We often have a bottle of diluted juice in our refrigerator. Diluted juice has a slightly sweet taste, but much less than full-strength juice. We also enjoy having sparkling water occasionally. It is very refreshing on a hot day.

Blended fruit drinks are a wonderful summertime treat. Children and adults love soy-milk fruit shakes and blended fruit drinks. Because these are such rich, sweet beverages, it is best to reserve them for special occasions.

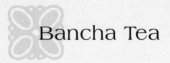

Bancha Tea

YIELD: 4 CUPS

4 cups water
1 tablespoon bancha twigs

Place water and twigs in teapot. Bring to boil and either turn off flame and let tea steep until color is deep golden brown; or bring to boil, turn flame to low, and simmer for about 10 minutes. The second version makes a stronger version than the first.

Other Available Beverages

The following beverages can be found in your natural foods store or grocery store.

Spring water—This is pure, nonpolluted water derived from a clean spring. For those people who don't have access to a spring, this water can be purchased in bottles from water companies, supermarkets, or health food stores.

Natural sparkling water—This is sometimes called seltzer water. It is carbonated water that may be purchased in bottles in supermarkets, liquor stores, or health food stores. Flavored, unsweetened, sparkling water may also be purchased with just a hint of lemon, lime, orange, cherry, or other fruit essences.

Apple juice or cider

Nonalcoholic beer—This beverage tastes like the real thing, but there is no alcohol and none of the alcohol side effects. It is especially refreshing on a hot summer day.

Instant Grain Coffee

YIELD: 1 CUP

1 cup water
1 teaspoon instant grain coffee

For one serving, heat water to boiling. Pour into a cup containing one teaspoon of grain coffee. Stir to dissolve and serve. For a stronger-tasting beverage, add more grain coffee.

Sparkling Water with Fruit Concentrate

YIELD: 1 CUP

1 cup sparkling water
1–2 teaspoons apple, cherry, raspberry, or other fruit concentrate

Stir concentrate into sparkling water and serve.

Summertime Coolers

A blender is necessary to prepare these tasty, refreshing treats for the hottest days of summer. Children especially find these enjoyable. Use your imagination when creating fruit combinations. Here are two examples:

YIELD: 1 SERVING

Apple-Strawberry Cooler
1 cup apple juice
½ cup strawberries
½–1 cup crushed ice

YIELD: 1 SERVING

Pear Cooler
1 cup apple juice
1 ripe pear
½–1 cup crushed ice

For each of these beverages, put ingredients in blender, adding ice gradually as you blend to achieve desired consistency.

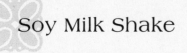

Soy Milk Shake

YIELD: 1 SERVING

6-ounce container of carob or vanilla soy milk
½–1 cup crushed ice

Put soy milk in blender and add ice gradually as you blend to achieve desired consistency.

Variations

- Add 1 level teaspoon of grain coffee to carob soy milk for a mocha shake.
- Add ½ cup fresh blueberries, ½ cup pitted cherries, or ½ cup strawberries to vanilla soy milk for a fruity shake.
- Add grain coffee or fruit to the blender and purée until smooth and thick.

Roasted Barley Tea (Mugi Cha)

YIELD: 4 CUPS

4 cups water
2 tablespoons roasted barley

Place water and barley in teapot. Bring to boil, lower heat, and simmer for 5 minutes for mild tea, or for 10–15 minutes for stronger flavor. This is a tasty beverage served hot or cool.

Appendix

MENU PLANS

As you read the recipes, you may have been surprised to see how much variety the macrobiotic diet offers. Following are menu plans for one week, and a meal plan for a holiday dinner. If you follow these plans, you can look forward to a delicious variety of filling foods at each meal.

Menu Plans		
Breakfast	*Lunch*	*Dinner*
Mochi Broiled Tofu Steamed Kale Bancha Tea	Tangy Rice Salad Nori Strips Cucumber with Umeboshi Vinegar Bancha Tea	Miso Soup Brown Rice with Barley Tempeh-Vegetable Combo Spring Salad Pecan-Oatmeal Cookies Grain Coffee

Apricot Soft Rice
Toasted Sunflower
   Seeds
Bancha Tea
	Arame Rice Triangles
	Tamari dip
	Leftover Tempeh—sliced,
	   and placed on rice cakes
	   with mustard and kraut
	Bancha Tea
		Miso Corn Soup
		Fettucine Lermano
		Garlic Tossed Salad
		Boiled Broccoli
		Bancha Tea

Menu Plans *(continued)*

Breakfast	*Lunch*	*Dinner*

Scrambled Tofu
Carrot Couscous
   Muffins
Bancha Tea
	Black-and-White Noodle
	   Salad
	Boiled Turnips
	Sweet Rice Corn Bread
	   with Apple Butter
	Bancha Tea
		Cream of Broccoli Soup
		Garlic-Miso Swordfish
		Boiled Long-Grain Brown Rice
		Marinated Daikon-Carrot Salad
		Steamed Buttercup Squash
		Apple Dumplings
		Grain Coffee

Variety Soft Rice
Leftover Squash
Bancha Tea
	Poppy-Lemon Rice
	Carrot Salad
	Rice Cakes with Sesame
	   Butter
	Bancha Tea
		Pinto Beans–Red Pepper Soup
		Crusty Millet Pizza with
		   Carrot Sauce
		Salad with Miso Dressing
		Olives
		Bancha Tea

Sweet Millet
Bancha Tea
	Barley Leek Soup
	Boiled Tofu on Sourdough
	   Bread and Mustard, Kraut,
	   and Grilled Onion
	Steamed Collard Greens
	   with Toasted Almonds
	Bancha Tea
		Sunchoke Vegetable Soup
		Medium-Grain Brown Rice
		Enchiladas
		Steamed Kale
		Chilled Peppers and Tofu Salad
		Couscous Apple Pie
		Grain Coffee

Scrambled Tofu
Rice and Onion
   Muffins (using
   leftover rice)
Bancha Tea
	Pine-Nut Rice Pancakes
	Steamed Carrott
	Bancha Tea
		Lentil Soup
		Baked Mushroom Grain Squares
		Steamed Watercress with
		   Sesame Seeds
		Quiche Nelson
		Grain Coffee

Breakfast	Lunch	Dinner
Ramen Pancake with Tofu Cream Dressing Bancha Tea	Miso-Lemon Bean Spread on Rice Cakes Umeboshi Salad Cabbage with Tofu Bancha Tea	Cream Tofu Soup Glazed Sesame Seitan Rolls Rice Pilaf Steamed Butternut Squash Umeboshi Salad Nutty Sweet Fruit Supreme Bancha Tea

Holiday Dinner

Navy Bean Seed Spread with Whole-Grain Crackers and Corn Chips (page 154)

Cream of Broccoli Soup (page 34)

Seitan Wellington (pages 92–93)

Garlic Tossed Salad (page 156)

Waldorf Salad Variation (pages 143–144)

Poppy-Lemon Rice (Page 52)

Boiled Carrots brushed with sesame oil, salt, and rice syrup and put under the broiler to glaze

Dill Pickles (pages 150–151)

Sticky Pecan Rolls (pages 186–187)

Apple Strudel (page 158)

Grain Coffee, Bancha Tea, Nonalcoholic Beer

Glossary

The following glossary describes macrobiotic foods, cooking methods, kitchen equipment, and ideas that may not be familiar to you. Words that have particular application to the relationship between diet and health are also included.

Agar-agar. A white gelatinous substance derived from a sea vegetable. Agar-agar is used in making aspics and kanten. *See also:* Kanten.

Amasake (Rice Milk). A sweetener or refreshing drink made from sweet rice and koji starter that is allowed to ferment into thick liquid. Hot amasake is a delicious beverage on cold autumn or winter nights.

Arame. A dark brown, spaghetti-like sea vegetable similar to hijiki. Rich in iron, calcium, and other minerals, arame is often used as a side dish.

Arrowroot. A starch flour processed from the root of an American native plant. It is used as a thickening agent, similar to cornstarch or kuzu, for making sauces, stews, and desserts.

Azuki Beans. Small, dark red beans. Especially good when cooked with kombu. This bean may also be referred to as *adzuki* or *aduki*.

Bancha Tea. Correctly named *kukicha,* bancha consists of the twigs and leaves from mature Japanese tea bushes. Bancha aids digestion, is high in calcium, and contains no chemical dyes. It makes an excellent breakfast or after-dinner beverage.

Barley, Pearl. A strain of barley native to China, pearl barley grows well in cold climates. It is good in stews and soups, or cooked with other grains. Pearl barley helps the body to eliminate animal fats.

Barley Malt. A thick, dark brown sweetener made from barley. Pure (100 percent) barley malt is used in making desserts, sweet-and-sour sauces, and in a variety of medicinal drinks.

Black Sesame Seeds. Small black seeds used occasionally as a garnish or to make black gomashio, a condiment. These seeds are different from the usual white or tan variety.

Bok Choy. A leafy, green vegetable with thick white stems that resemble stalks. Bok choy is used mostly in summer cooking. It is sometimes called *pok choy*.

Brown Rice. Unpolished rice with only its tough outer husk removed. It comes in three main varieties: short, medium, and long grain. Short-grain brown rice contains the best balance of minerals, protein, and carbohydrates, but the other types may also be used on occasion. *See also:* Sweet Brown Rice.

Brown Rice Miso. Miso made from soybeans, brown rice, and sea salt, fermented for approximately twelve months. Used in making soups and seasoning vegetable dishes.

Brown Rice Vinegar. A very mild and delicate vinegar made from fermented brown rice or sweet brown rice. Brown rice vinegar is not as acid-forming in the body as apple cider vinegar.

Buckwheat. A cereal plant native to Siberia, buckwheat has been a staple food in many European countries for several centuries. It is frequently eaten in the form of kasha, whole groats, or soba noodles.

Burdock. A hardy plant that grows wild throughout the United States. The long, dark burdock root is delicious in soups, stews, and sea vegetable dishes, or sautéed with carrots. It is highly valued in macrobiotic cooking for its strengthening qualities. The Japanese name is *gobo*.

Chinese Cabbage. A large, leafy vegetable with pale green tops and thick white stems. Sometimes called *nappa,* this juicy, slightly sweet vegetable is good in soups and stews, vegetable dishes, and pickled.

Couscous. A partially refined and quick-cooking cracked wheat that has a flavor similar to Cream of Wheat.

Daikon. A long, white radish. Besides making a delicious side dish, daikon helps dissolve stagnant fat and mucous deposits that have accumulated in the body. Freshly grated raw daikon is especially helpful in the digestion of oily foods.

Dried Daikon. Daikon sold in dried and shredded form. Dried daikon is especially good cooked with kombu and seasoned with tamari soy sauce. Soaking dried daikon before use brings out its natural sweetness.

Dried Tofu. Tofu that has been naturally dehydrated by freezing. Used in soups, stews, vegetable and sea vegetable dishes, dried tofu contains less fat than regular tofu. *See also:* tofu.

Dulse. A reddish-purple sea vegetable used in soups, salads, and vegetable dishes. Dulse is high in protein, iron, vitamin A, iodine, and phosphorus. Most of the dulse sold in America comes from Canada, Maine, and Massachusetts.

Fiber. The indigestible portion of whole foods; particularly, the bran of whole grains and outer skins of legumes, vegetables, and fruits. Fiber facilitates the passage of waste through the intestines. Foods that are refined, processed, or peeled are low in fiber.

Fu. A dried wheat-gluten product. Available in thin sheets or thick round cakes, fu is a satisfying high-protein food used in soups, stews, and vegetable dishes.

Ginger. A spicy, pungent, golden-colored root, used as a garnish or seasoning in cooking and for various beverages. Also used in making external home remedies such as the ginger compress.

Gluten (Wheat). The sticky substance that remains after the bran has been kneaded and rinsed from whole-wheat flour. Gluten is used to make seitan and fu.

Gomashio. Also known as *sesame salt.* Gomashio is a table condiment made from roasted, ground sesame seeds and sea salt. It is good sprinkled on brown rice and other whole grains.

Grain Coffee. A nonstimulating, caffeine-free coffee substitute made from roasted grains, beans, and roots. Ingredients are combined in different ways to create a variety of different flavors. Used like instant coffee.

Green Nori Flakes. A sea vegetable condiment made from a certain type of nori, different from the packaged variety. The flakes are rich in iron, calcium, and vitamin A. They can be sprinkled on whole grains, vegetables, salads, and other dishes.

Hatcho Miso. Miso made from soybeans and sea salt and fermented for a minimum of two years. It has a mild salt taste and may be used from time to time in making soup stocks and condiments, and for seasoning vegetable dishes. This dark, rich miso is especially good in cold weather.

Hijiki. A dark-brown sea vegetable that turns black when dried. It has a spaghetti-like consistency, a stronger taste than arame, and is very high in calcium and protein. The hijiki sold in the United States is imported from Japan or harvested off the coast of Maine.

Hokkaido Pumpkin. There are two varieties of Hokkaido pumpkin. One has a deep orange color and the other has a light green skin similar to Hubbard squash. Both varieties are very sweet and have a tough outer skin.

Japanese Black Beans. A special type of soybean grown in Japan. They can be used to alleviate problems of the reproductive organs. In cooking, these black beans are used in soups and side dishes.

Kanten. A jelled dessert made from agar-agar. It can include seasonal fruits such as melons, apples, berries, peaches, and pears, or amasake, azuki beans, and other items. Usually served chilled, it is a refreshing alternative to conventional gelatin.

Kasha. Buckwheat groats that are roasted prior to boiling. Kasha is a traditional European and Russian food.

Kayu. Cereal grain cooked with five to ten times as much water as grain, for a long period of time. Kayu is ready when it is soft and creamy.

Kelp. A large family of sea vegetables that grow profusely off both coasts of the United States. Kelp is widely available at natural foods stores, packaged whole, granulated, or powdered. It is an excellent source of minerals, including iodine.

Koji. A grain, usually semi-polished or polished rice, inoculated with bacteria and used to begin the fermentation process in a variety of foods, including miso, amasake, tamari, natto, and sake.

Kombu. A wide, thick, dark green sea vegetable that is rich in minerals. Kombu is often cooked with beans and vegetables. A single piece may be reused several times to flavor soup stock.

Kuzu. A white starch made from the root of the wild kuzu plant. In this country, the plant densely populates the southern states, where it is called *kudzu*. It is used in making soups, sauces, desserts, and medicinal beverages.

Lotus. The root and seeds of a water lily that is brown skinned with a hollow, chambered, off-white inside. Lotus is especially good for the sinuses and lungs. The seeds are used in grain, bean, and sea vegetable dishes.

Macrobiotics. An approach to balanced living, based on a balanced diet, moderate exércise, harmony with the environment, and an understanding of the philosophic principles of yin and yang. George Ohsawa was the first to recognize how these traditional concepts could be applied to modern living.

Millet. A small, yellow grain that comes in many varieties, with pearled millet being the most common. Millet is used in soups, vegetable dishes, casseroles, and as a cereal.

Mirin. A cooking wine made from whole-grain sweet rice. Be careful when purchasing mirin, as many varieties on the market have been processed with refined grain and additives.

Miso. A protein-rich fermented soybean paste made from ingredients such as soybeans, barley, and brown or white rice. Miso is used in soup stocks and as a seasoning. When consumed on a regular basis, it aids circulation and digestion. Mugi miso is usually best for daily use, but other varieties may be used occasionally. Quick or short-term misos, which are fermented for several weeks, are less suitable for frequent use; their salt content is higher than that of the longer-term varieties such as mugi and hatcho miso. *See also:* Hatcho Miso; Natto Miso; Onazaki Miso; Red Miso; White Miso; Yellow Miso.

Miso, Puréed. Miso that has been reduced to a smooth, creamy texture that will allow it to blend easily with other ingredients. To purée miso, place it in a bowl or suribachi and add enough water or broth to make a smooth paste. Blend with a wooden pestle or spoon.

Mochi. A heavy rice cake or dumpling made from cooked, pounded sweet brown rice. Mochi is especially good for lactating mothers, as it promotes the production of breast milk. Mochi can be prepared at home or purchased ready-made; it makes an excellent snack.

Mugicha. A tea made from roasted unhulled barley and water. Mugicha may be served hot, or as a refreshing chilled beverage in the summer.

Mugi Miso. A miso made from barley, soybeans, and sea salt, fermented for about eighteen to twenty-four months. This flavorful miso can be used on a daily basis year-round to make soup stocks, condiments, and pickles, and to season vegetable or bean dishes. Mugi miso is generally suitable for use by individuals with serious illness.

Mu Tea. Tea made from a blend of traditional, nonstimulating herbs. A warming and strengthening beverage, mu tea is especially beneficial for the female reproductive organs. Two popular varieties of mu tea are #9 and #16.

Natto. Soybeans that have been cooked, mixed with beneficial enzymes, and allowed to ferment for twenty-four hours. Natto is high in easy-to-digest protein and vitamin B_{12}.

Natto Miso. A condiment made from soybeans, barley, kombu, and ginger; not actually a miso.

Natural Foods. Foods that are not processed or treated with artificial additives or preservatives. Some natural foods are partially refined using traditional methods.

Nigari. A coagulant made from sea salt, used in making tofu.

Nishime. A method of cooking in which different combinations of vegetables, sea vegetables, or soybean products are slow-cooked with a small amount of water and tamari soy sauce. Also referred to as *waterless cooking*.

Nori. Thin black or dark purple sheets of dried sea vegetable. Nori is often roasted over a flame until it turns green. It is used as a garnish, wrapped around rice balls in making sushi, or cooked with tamari soy sauce as a condiment. It is rich in vitamins and minerals. It is sometimes called *laver*.

Oden. A dish in which root vegetables, sea vegetables, soybean products, and sometimes fish are simmered together for a long time. Many combinations of ingredients are used in making this excellent winter stew.

Ohagi. Glutenous patties made from cooked, pounded sweet rice rolled in or coated with roasted and ground sesame seeds, roasted ground nuts, puréed azuki beans and raisins, etc. Frequently eaten as a dessert.

Onazaki Miso. A miso made from white rice, soybeans, and sea salt. Lighter in color than mugi and hatcho miso, and slightly saltier, onazaki miso has a rich flavor. It is used occasionally in making soup stocks and for seasoning vegetable dishes.

Organic Foods. Foods grown and harvested without the use of synthetically compounded chemical fertilizers, pesticides, herbicides, and fungicides.

Pressed Salad. Very thinly sliced or shredded fresh vegetables, combined with a pickling agent such as sea salt, umeboshi, brown rice vinegar, or tamari soy sauce, and placed in a pickle press. In the pickling process, many of the enzymes and vitamins are retained while the vegetables become easier to digest.

Red Miso. A salty-tasting short-term fermented miso, made from soybeans and sea salt. Suitable for occasional use by individuals who are in good health. Also called *aka miso*.

Refined Oil. Salad or cooking oil that has been chemically extracted and processed to maximize yield and extend shelf life. Refining strips an oil of its color, flavor, and aroma, and reduces its nutritive value.

Rice Balls. Rice shaped into balls or triangles, usually with a piece of umeboshi in the center, and wrapped in toasted nori or shiso leaves to completely cover. For variety, different ingredients may be used as filling or for a coating. Rice balls are good for snacks, lunches, picnics, and traveling.

Rice Syrup. *See* Yinnie syrup.

Sake. Japanese rice wine containing about 15 percent alcohol, often used in cooking.

Sea Salt. Salt obtained from evaporated seawater, as opposed to rock salt mined from inland beds. Sea salt is either sun baked or kiln baked. High in trace minerals, it contains no sugar or chemical additives.

Sea Vegetables. Any variety of marine plants used as food. Sea vegetables are a prime source of vitamins, minerals, and trace elements in the macrobiotic diet.

Seitan. Wheat gluten cooked in tamari soy sauce, kombu, and water. Seitan can be made at home or purchased ready-made at many natural foods stores. It is high in protein and has a chewy texture, making it an ideal meat substitute.

Sesame Butter. A nut butter obtained by roasting and grinding brown sesame seeds until smooth and creamy. It is used like peanut butter or in salad dressings and sauces.

Shiitake. Mushrooms imported dried from Japan and available freshly grown in some parts of the United States. Either type can be used to flavor soup stocks or vegetable dishes, and dried shiitake can also be used in medicinal preparations. These mushrooms help the body to discharge excess animal fats.

Shiso. A red, pickled leaf. The plant is known in English as the *beefstake plant*. Shiso leaves are used to color umeboshi plums and as a condiment. Sometimes spelled *chiso*.

Shoyu. *See* Tamari and Tamari Soy Sauce.

Soba. Noodles made from buckwheat flour or a combination of buckwheat and (whole) wheat flour. Soba can be served in broth, in salads, or with vegetables. In the summer, soba noodles are great chilled.

Somen. Very thin white or whole-wheat Japanese noodles. Thinner than soba and other whole-grain noodles, somen are often served during the summer.

Sprouted Wheat Bread. A whole-grain bread made from soaked wheat that is sprouted and baked. Sprouted wheat bread does not contain flour, salt, or oil, and is very sweet and moist.

Suribachi. A special serrated, glazed clay bowl. Used with a pestle, called a surikogi, for grinding and puréeing foods. An essential item in the macrobiotic kitchen, the suribachi can be used in a variety of ways to make condiments, spreads, dressings, baby foods, nut butters, and medicinal preparations.

Surikogi. A wooden pestle that is used with a suribachi. Used to make gomashio, sea vegetable powders, and other condiments, and to mash foods to obtain a creamy consistency.

Sushi. Rice rolled with vegetables, fish, or pickles, wrapped in nori, and sliced in rounds. Sushi is becoming increasingly popular throughout the United States. The most healthful sushi is made with brown rice and other natural ingredients.

Sushi Mat. Very thin strips of bamboo that are fastened together with cotton thread so that they can be rolled tightly yet allow air to pass through freely. These mats are used in rolling sushi, and also to cover freshly cooked foods or leftovers.

Sweet Brown Rice. A sweeter-tasting, more glutenous variety of brown rice. Sweet brown rice is used in mochi, ohagi, dumplings, baby foods, vinegar, and amasake. It is often used in cooking for festive occasions.

Tahini. A nut butter obtained by grinding hulled white sesame seeds until smooth and creamy. It is used like sesame butter.

Takuan. Daikon that is pickled in rice bran and sea salt. It is named after the Buddhist priest who invented this particular pickling method. Sometimes spelled *takuwan*.

Tamari and Tamari Soy Sauce. Tamari soy sauce is traditional, naturally made soy sauce, as distinguished from chemically processed varieties. Original or "real" tamari is the liquid poured off during the process of making hatcho miso. The best-quality tamari soy sauce is naturally fermented for over a year and is made from whole soybeans, wheat, and sea salt. Tamari soy sauce is sometimes referred to as *shoyu*.

Taro. A type of potato with a thick, dark brown, hairy skin. It is eaten as a vegetable or used in the preparation of plasters for medicinal purposes.

Tekka. A condiment made from hatcho miso, sesame oil, burdock, lotus root, carrot, and ginger root. Tekka is sautéed over a low flame for several hours. It is dark brown in color and very rich in iron.

Tempeh. A traditional soy food, made from split soybeans, water, and beneficial bacteria, and allowed to ferment for several hours. Tempeh is eaten in Indonesia and Sri Lanka as a staple food. Rich in easy-to-digest protein and vitamin B_{12}, tempeh is available prepackaged in some natural foods stores.

Tempura. A method of cooking in which seasoned vegetables and fish or seafood are coated with batter and deep-fried in unrefined oil. Tempura is often served with soup and pickles.

Tofu. Soybean curd, made from soybeans and nigari. Tofu is a protein-rich soyfood used in soups, vegetable dishes, dressings, etc. *See also:* Dried Tofu.

Udon. Japanese-style noodles made from wheat, whole wheat, or whole wheat and unbleached white flour. Udon have a lighter flavor than soba (buckwheat) noodles and can be used in the same ways.

Umeboshi. Salty, pickled plums that stimulate the appetite and digestion and aid in maintaining an alkaline blood quality. Shiso leaves impart a reddish color and natural flavoring to the plums during pickling. Umeboshi can be used whole or in the form of a paste.

Umeboshi Vinegar. A salty, sour vinegar made from umeboshi plums. Diluted with water, it is used in sweet-and-sour sauces, salads, salad dressings, etc.

Unrefined Oil. Pressed and/or solvent-extracted vegetable oil that retains the original color, flavor, aroma, and nutritional value of the natural substance.

Wakame. A long, thin, green sea vegetable used in making a variety of dishes. High in protein, iron, and magnesium, wakame has a sweet taste and delicate textures. It is especially good in miso soup.

Washabi. A light green Japanese horseradish that is used in sushi or traditionally with raw fish (sashimi). Wasabi is a very hot spice.

Wheat Gluten. *See* Gluten (Wheat).

Wheat Berries. The grains of whole wheat are often called wheat berries. They are used to make whole-wheat flours and noodles. They can also be soaked and pressure-cooked with brown rice or other whole grains.

White Miso. A sweet-tasting short-term fermented miso made from white rice, soybeans, and sea salt. Used in making soup stocks and sometimes in vegetable dishes. Suitable for occasional use by individuals who are in good health. Also called *shiro miso*.

Whole Foods. The edible portions of foods as they come from nature, unprocessed, nutritionally complete, and without chemical additives. Whole foods are not refined at all.

Wild Rice. A wild grass that grows in water and is harvested by hand. Eaten traditionally by Native Americans in Minnesota and other areas. These long, dark, thin grains are available at many natural foods stores.

Yang. In macrobiotics, energy or movement that has a centripetal or inward direction. One of the two antagonistic yet complementary forces that together describe all phenomena, yang is traditionally symbolized by a triangle ($\triangle$). *See also* Yin.

Yellow Miso. A short-term fermented miso made from white rice, soybeans, and sea salt. This miso has a salty but very mellow flavor and is used in making soups, sauces, and vegetable dishes. It is suitable for occasional use by individuals who are in good health.

Yin. In macrobiotics, energy or movement that has a centrifugal or outward direction and results in expansion. One of the two antagonistic yet complementary forces that together describe all phenomena, yin is traditionally symbolized by an inverted triangle ($\triangledown$). *See also:* Yang.

Yinnie Syrup. A sweet, thick syrup, made from brown rice and barley, that is used in dessert cooking. This complex-carbohydrate sweetener is preferable to simple sugars such as honey, maple syrup, and molasses, because the simple sugars are metabolized too quickly. Also called *rice syrup*.

Resources

SPROUT HOUSE AND MACROBIOTICS
15233 Kercheval Street
Grosse Pointe Park, MI 48230
(313) 331-3200

GEORGE OHSAWA MACROBIOTIC FOUNDATION
P.O. Box 3998
Chico, CA 95927-3998
(800) 232-2372
www.gomf.macrobiotic.net

WILD OATS
For store locations across the country.
www.wildoats.com

THE KUSHI INSTITUTE
P.O. Box 7
Becket, MA 01223
(800) 975-8744
www.kushiinstitute.org

SPRING STREET NATURAL RESTAURANT
62 Spring Street
New York, NY 10014
(212) 966-0290

OAK FEED NATURAL FOOD MARKET AND RESTAURANT
3155 Oak Avenue
Miami, FL 33133
(305) 448-7595

MENDOCINO SEA VEGETABLE COMPANY
P.O. Box 1265
Mendocino, CA 95460
(707) 895-2996
www.seaweed.net
info@seaweed.net

MARGARET LAWSON
THE MACROBIOTIC CENTER OF DALLAS
For cooking class scheduling, or bed-and-breakfast availability:
P.O. Box 79-6731
Dallas, TX 75379
(903) 786-9100
www.macrobioticcenter.com
macro@airmail.net

IONIA, INC.
54932 Burdock Road
Kasilof, AK 99610
(907) 262-2824

THE MACROBIOTIC CENTER OF NEW YORK
(212) 505-1010

Index